Dwarfism Arts and Advocacy

With an unequivocal commitment to the creation of new insights which challenge the dynamics of disablism, this collection provides a rare assemblage of insider knowledge on dwarfism, identity, and the arts. Rooted firmly in the initial principles of Disability Studies, with its centering of disabled people's situated knowledges, whilst benefitting from more recent developments in Cultural Disability Studies, Pritchard, a leading figure in studies of dwarfism, has gathered the stories and arguments of an extensive range of people with dwarfism. All these contributors are well-positioned to provide a diverse body of accounts relating to dwarfism, setting personal aspects of life within wider social and cultural structures and contexts. All, together, this wide range of threads weave a rich tapestry, making a compelling statement for change in arts practice and wider cultural attitudes to dwarfism.
—*Alison Wilde*, **author of Film, Comedy, and Disability: Understanding Humour and Genre in Cinematic Constructions of Impairment and Disability**

Dwarfism Arts and Advocacy finally gives voice to the challenges of navigating the entertainment world as an artist with dwarfism. Whether it be in film, television, visual arts or art education, the authors of this collective share insights into the myriad of obstacles that stand in the way of forging a dignified artistic path in an ableist space. Every artist struggles with identity, individuality, and inconceivable odds. However, these artists explain in such vulnerable detail, the challenge of trying to destabilise the historical narrative of the dwarf in art and culture. It's not a pretty past. And the struggle to create new imagery, representation and dignity against centuries of ridicule and contempt is powerful. This is a must read for anyone who believes in the expansion of voices and perspectives in the art world.
—*Mark Povinelli*, **Star of** *Nightmare Alley*; **Past President of Little People of America**

The chapters in this book represent a wide range of voices from artists, performers, writers, advocates, and across diverse platforms including podcasters and bloggers, all within the dwarfism community from around the world. Each contributor shares their view and experience in relation to the challenges, frustrations, and barriers they have faced from society and portrayed within the arts, media, and film industries, each advocating for societal change to challenge the attitudes associated with dwarfism within the arts and media. It's evident that this book aims to bring crucial awareness and understanding to the challenges faced by individuals with dwarfism in life as well as in various industries, particularly in the arts, media, and film. By amplifying their voices and experiences this book has the potential to spark meaningful conversations and drive positive change in how dwarfism is represented and perceived in society. [...] Whether you're a person with dwarfism, friend or family member or a member of the wider community, whoever you are you will benefit from the insights and perspectives shared within these pages. This book is not just an educational resource it's a "call to action" for recognition of the need for greater inclusion, acknowledgement, and true-life representation of people with dwarfism across the arts, media, and film industries.

—*Maree Jenner*, **Vice President, SSPA**

Dwarfism Arts and Advocacy: Creating Our Own Positive Identity

EDITED BY

ERIN PRITCHARD

Liverpool Hope University, UK

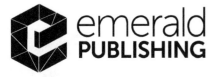

United Kingdom – North America – Japan – India – Malaysia – China

Emerald Publishing Limited
Emerald Publishing, Floor 5, Northspring, 21-23 Wellington Street, Leeds LS1 4DL

First edition 2024

Editorial matter and selection © 2024 Erin Pritchard.
Individual chapters © 2024 The authors.
Published under exclusive licence by Emerald Publishing Limited.

Reprints and permissions service
Contact: www.copyright.com

No part of this book may be reproduced, stored in a retrieval system, transmitted in any form or by any means electronic, mechanical, photocopying, recording or otherwise without either the prior written permission of the publisher or a licence permitting restricted copying issued in the UK by The Copyright Licensing Agency and in the USA by The Copyright Clearance Center. Any opinions expressed in the chapters are those of the authors. Whilst Emerald makes every effort to ensure the quality and accuracy of its content, Emerald makes no representation implied or otherwise, as to the chapters' suitability and application and disclaims any warranties, express or implied, to their use.

British Library Cataloguing in Publication Data
A catalogue record for this book is available from the British Library

ISBN: 978-1-83753-923-9 (Print)
ISBN: 978-1-83753-922-2 (Online)
ISBN: 978-1-83753-924-6 (Epub)

INVESTOR IN PEOPLE

Contents

About the Editor ix

About the Contributors xi

Acknowledgements xv

Introduction 1
Erin Pritchard

Chapter 1   Curating New Perspectives: How My Dwarfism Led Me to Disability Art 11
Amanda Cachia

Chapter 2   Little Big Woman: Condescension – Sculpting the Oppositional Gaze 25
Debra Keenahan

Chapter 3   Where Are the Creative Opportunities for People With Dwarfism Lived Experience in Participatory Arts Funding? 37
Steph Robson

Chapter 4   It's Behind You: How Equity and an Education Made Me More Than Just a Suit Filler 51
Alice Lambert and Erin Pritchard

Chapter 5   Midgitte Bardot: Using Drag Performance to Challenge People's Perceptions and Attitudes of Dwarfism 63
Tamm Reynolds and Erin Pritchard

Chapter 6 The Path to Success Is Long and Winding: Challenging Stereotypes and Fighting for Disability Equality in the Entertainment Industry 75
Danny Woodburn and Erin Pritchard

Chapter 7 Get the Balance Right: The Change in How People With Dwarfism Are Depicted From Limited, Damaging and Negative to Realistic, Creative and Positive 89
Simon Minty

Chapter 8 Creating Our Own Path: The Easterseals Disability Film Challenge 101
Nic Novicki and Erin Pritchard

Chapter 9 Dwarfism Advocacy: A Life Tenure 107
Angela Muir Van Etten

Chapter 10 Exploring Dwarfism Representation in Social Media: Intentionality and Advocacy as a Digital Content Creator 121
Kara B. Ayers

Chapter 11 Podcasts as a Platform for Advocacy 131
Jillian Curwin

Chapter 12 The Patchwork Representation We Too Often Miss 139
Sam Drummond

Chapter 13 'Would You Befriend Me, Date Me, Hire Me if I Hadn't Had My Bones Broken & Stretched to Look More Like Yours?' 145
Emily Sullivan Sanford

Epilogue 161
Erin Pritchard

Index 167

About the Editor

Erin Pritchard is a Senior Lecturer in Disability Studies at Liverpool Hope University and a core member of the Centre for Culture and Disability Studies. Her recent book, *Midgetism: The Exploitation and Discrimination of People with Dwarfism*, explores problematic representations and societal attitudes associated with dwarfism. Her work centres on how cultural representations of dwarfism influence the social understanding of the condition. She is currently a consultant for Disney, specialising in representations of dwarfism.

About the Contributors

Kara B. Ayers is an Associate Professor and the Associate Director of the University of Cincinnati Centre for Excellence in Developmental Disabilities at Cincinnati Children's Hospital Medical Centre. Dr Ayers is trained as a Psychologist and leads the National Centre for Disability, Equity and Intersectionality, where she works to advance disability justice through an intersectional lens. Dr Ayers' research interests include disability in media, disability ethics and parenting with a disability. In addition to her scholarly work, Dr Ayers has served as a consultant for several major media companies related to portrayals and representation of disability.

Amanda Cachia has an established career profile as a curator, consultant, writer and art historian who specializes in disability art activism. She is the Assistant Professor and Assistant Director of the Masters of Arts in Arts Leadership Graduate Program at the Kathrine G. McGovern College of the Arts at the University of Houston. She is a 2023 grantee of the Creative Capital | Andy Warhol Foundation Arts Writers Grant for her second monograph, *Hospital Aesthetics: Rescripting Medical Images of Disability*. Her first book, *The Agency of Access: Contemporary Disability Art and Institutional Critique*, is forthcoming with Temple University Press (2024). Cachia is also the editor of *Curating Access: Disability Art Activism and Creative Accommodation* (2022) published by Routledge, which includes over 40 international contributors. She has a PhD in Art History, Theory & Criticism from the University of California San Diego. Cachia has curated approximately 50 exhibitions, many of which have traveled to cities across the USA, England, Australia and Canada.

Jillian Curwin is a writer, content creator and advocate for dwarfism and disability awareness based in New York City. She has written articles for Betches Media talking about disability representation in fashion and entertainment along with highlighting current events in the disability space. In addition, she has consulted with brands and organisations about disability inclusion. She is the host of the podcast *Always Looking Up* where she talks to little people, disabled people, those that are disabled-adjacent and allies about living in a world that was not necessarily designed for them.

Sam Drummond is a lawyer, author and disability advocate. Sam studied Arts and Law at Monash University in Melbourne, Australia. He began his career as a broadcaster and producer on community, commercial and public radio, before moving onto a career in law. His debut book, Broke, is a memoir about navigating the world through disability, downward mobility and unconventional families.

Debra Keenahan is an artist, writer, psychologist and disability advocate. She has a PhD in Psychology on Dehumanisation and another in visual arts on Critical Disability Aesthetics. Having achondroplasia dwarfism, Debra brings lived experience to understanding the dynamics of interactions of exclusion. As a multi-discipline artist, Debra's video work was selected for the Cannes Short Film Festival 2022 and her one-woman theatre work 'Othering', featured in the Sydney Festival 2023. Debra has authored numerous books and articles and has acted as a consultant on disability access to the National Gallery of Australia and NAVA (National Association of Visual Artists).

Alice Lambert is a Performance Artist and Actor as well as a Teacher of Drama and Contemporary Dance. Alice graduated from the University of East Anglia in 2023 with a degree in English Literature and Drama. She has appeared in numerous theatre plays and films, including Mary Poppins Returns (2018). Alice is passionate about raising awareness and challenging stereotypes about dwarfism through her work.

Simon Minty is a disability trainer and consultant. He advises major organisations on disabled people's inclusion in employment and customer interactions; plus broadcasters and creatives on the representation of people with dwarfism and other conditions. He is on the board of the National Theatre and Motability Operations plc. Simon co-hosts the podcast The Way We Roll and is a former co-host of BBC Access All. He co-founded the comedy troupe, Abnormally Funny People. He has a BSc in Philosophy and Sociology and postgraduate diploma in Disability Management at Work, both from City, University of London.

Nic Novicki graduated from the American Academy of Dramatic Arts, Temple University Fox School of Business, the school of Film and Television, and UCB Theatre. He is an actor, comedian and producer. He has appeared in numerous television shows including Boardwalk Empire and The Sopranos. He has also appeared in several movies, including Spider-Man: Across the Spider-Verse. He has produced several feature films, television pilots and web series for companies including Sony and Universal. Nic has also performed stand-up for AXS Gotham Comedy Live. He is the founder of the Easterseals Disability Film Challenge.

Tamm Reynolds is a solo artist also known as Midgitte Bardot (who is the most glamourous coping mechanism in the world). They have been performing across the UK cabaret, live art, drag, theatre and club spaces since 2016. Now, working on a solo show after two previous work-in-progresses (2022 & 2023), alongside starring in Royal Court's Sound of the Underground (written by Travis Alabanza and directed by Debbie Hannan) in a winter run in 2023. In 2023, she featured in a special issue of Vogue.

Steph Robson, aka *Hello, Little Lady*, is a creative practitioner and artist. Since graduating from Sunderland University with an MA in Radio (Production and Management) in 2006, she has been writing and making art to platform and give a voice to the lived experience of people with dwarfism. Her debut photographic exhibition 'You're Just Little' in 2018 revealed the obstacles, challenges and societal assumptions that dwarf people face every day. Her work explores the themes of accessibility, othering and the tensions between disability and society.

Emily Sullivan Sanford is a writer, blogger and speaker specialising in disability, beauty standards, bioethics and intersectional oppressions. Based in Berlin, she leads diversity workshops and collaborates with online platforms that question media representation of minorities. In the United States, she has worked with the Children of Difference Foundation and the Hastings Centre, a bioethics think tank. Her writing has been published by Salon, Feministing, John Hopkins University Press and others. She lives with her family in Berlin.

Angela Muir Van Etten graduated with law degrees from the University of Auckland in New Zealand and the University of Maryland in America. Van Etten retired from a diverse career as a barrister and solicitor, writing and editing law books for Thomson Reuters, writing for a nonprofit Christian organisation, and advocating for people with disabilities. As a dwarf, Van Etten was propelled to serve as national president of dwarfism organisations in New Zealand and the United States, advocate on dwarfism and disability issues and to write a dwarfism memoir trilogy and weekly blog.

Danny Woodburn is a journeyman actor and a graduate of Temple University Theatre and Film with over 150 TV appearances (*Seinfeld, Bookie*) and 30 films (*Watchmen, Death to Smoochy*). As a person with dwarfism, he advocates for all performers with disability (PWD), serving on SAG-AFTRA's PWD Committee, changing contract language, studio DEI policy and shifting the industry to acknowledge disabled performers in inclusion and access practices by launching an awareness campaign in the Huffington Post Op-Ed, 'If You Don't Really Mean Inclusion – Shut the F%&# Up!', *The Ruderman White Paper on Employment of People With Disability in TV*, and articles in *The Hollywood Reporter, Variety, The Guardian, Forbes, WSJ, The Philadelphia Inquirer*.

Acknowledgements

As the editor, my biggest appreciation goes to all of the authors within this book, not just for their contributions but also for all of the hard work they do in challenging harmful stereotypes of dwarfism.

I would like to thank Professor David Bolt for his support, especially for his valuable feedback. I would also like to thank other colleagues in Disability Studies at Liverpool Hope University, including Ella Houston and Claire Penketh, as well as colleagues outside of the subject, such as Jody Crutchley.

Introduction

Erin Pritchard (Senior Lecturer in Disability Studies)
Liverpool Hope University, UK

When you think of a person with dwarfism, what image springs to mind? Now, hold onto that image and consider how you are expected to respond to it. Is your response laughter, amusement or maybe curiosity? Do you even see them as human or just a novelty for the entertainment of others? For people who have never met a person with dwarfism, and that will be the majority given the rarity of the condition, their point of reference will be a character with dwarfism they have seen in a fairy tale, a film, television show or perhaps someone on social media. A quick Google search of the term 'dwarf' brings up a mixture of numerous images of *Snow White and the Seven Dwarfs* and mythical dwarfs complete with long beard, axe and viking helmet. The former characters have been purposely constructed to signify the supposed inferiority of people with dwarfism. The latter images 'combine physical attributes associated with dwarfism and longstanding folk motifs about the supernatural' (Mock, 2020, p. 155). These are not natural or realistic representations of dwarfism but rather are socially and culturally constructed to assume that people with dwarfism are not fully human but rather something different and often amusing. Very few people would question cultural constructions of dwarfism but assume instead that is how we are naturally or that we are accepting to these representations.

How people are represented, particularly minority groups, is important to consider. Representations are an act of power, as they influence how people are perceived and subsequently treated. Dwarfism is a condition that most people know of, yet know very little about. The media reduces people with dwarfism to figures of fun who have to rely on midget entertainment, as their dwarfism somehow makes them incapable of any other form of employment. Growing up, I was only ever exposed to the metanarrative of dwarfism, and yet I knew I was not like the dwarfs I saw in the media. It was in Betty Adelson's (2005b) book, 'The Lives of Dwarfs: Their Journey from Public Curiosity Toward Social Liberation' where I first learnt about a myriad of very successful people with dwarfism, working in numerous occupations. Before this, the only books I saw people with dwarfism in were fairy tales and books about freak shows.

Throughout history, representations of dwarfism have been controlled by average-sized people, in what Professor David Bolt terms the metanarrative of disability. The metanarrative for disability can be defined as 'the grand story in relation to which people who have impairments often find themselves defined' (Bolt, 2019, p. 114). The metanarrative of dwarfism constructs people with dwarfism as entertaining figures of fun (Pritchard, 2021; Watson, 2020). General society, including children, learn about dwarfism through cultural representations of the condition, popular within the media, including films and television shows (Pritchard, 2023). These representations have created a distorted view of dwarfism which contributes to the abuse people with dwarfism experience within society (Ellis, 2018; Pritchard, 2021; Tan, 2021).

Bolt (2021) points out that the metanarrative of disability is favoured over personal narratives. What is frustrating is that a minority of midget entertainers have aided in perpetuating ableist stereotypes of dwarfism. I have previously reclaimed the word midget to emphasise how some forms of entertainment exploit and reinforce discriminatory representations of dwarfism (See Pritchard, 2023). As a result, people with dwarfism who partake in this form of entertainment are referred to as midget entertainers. What is problematic is that those who continue to partake in derogatory entertainment, including midget tossing, are given a more prominent platform to defend these ableist perceptions of dwarfism (Pritchard, 2023). Thus, we cannot rely on equality to appear; we need to fight for it.

A key aspect of challenging the metanarrative is recognising the importance of disability voice. Allowing those who advocate for a more positive representation of dwarfism to share personal narratives of the work they do aids in challenging long-held beliefs about dwarfism. If we want equality, then the first step is to challenge the metanarrative of dwarfism, which is informed by ableist notions of the condition. What society seems to be unaware of is that there are a growing number of people with dwarfism who are pushing against the metanarrative of dwarfism. They are advocates with dwarfism who are using various platforms to raise awareness.

Disability Arts and Advocacy

Disability arts and the media are important tools in challenging problematic stereotypes of disability, as well as giving disabled people a platform for creating their own representations. Disability arts offer disabled people the opportunity to expose disabling barriers within society (Allan, 2005). While numerous work has exposed and challenged problematic representations of dwarfism (see Ellis, 2018; Haberer, 2010; Mock, 2020; Pritchard, 2021, 2023; Pritchard & Kruse, 2020; Tyrrell, 2020; Watson, 2020), there is limited work exploring the advocacy work being done by people with dwarfism within the arts and media. The aim of this book is to challenge problematic stereotypes and attitudes associated with dwarfism in the arts and media by providing artists and activists with dwarfism a platform to showcase and explain their work.

This book was borne from my frustrations with the lack of representation of dwarfism in disability arts. That is not to say that there were no artists with dwarfism, but that disability arts is dominated by a particular representation. While I knew of some great artists with dwarfism involved in disability arts, I felt that there was a need to provide more of a collective voice to challenge the metanarrative of dwarfism. However, as this book developed, I realised that it was important to include other people with dwarfism who are utilising other forms of media, such as podcasts and blogs, to advocate for a more true-to-life representation of dwarfism.

I choose to only include people with dwarfism whose work does not promote derogatory representations of dwarfism. Forms of derogatory dwarf entertainment include anything which constructs people with dwarfism as inferior. Those who partake in midget entertainment, which I argue is an ableist form of entertainment used to keep people with dwarfism within an inferior place in society, are already given a big enough platform. Because midget entertainers are perpetuating ableist stereotypes of dwarfism, they are often defended and given a voice by mainstream media. For example, I have come across numerous news stories about derogatory midget entertainment, such as hiring out a midget entertainer for a celebratory event. These stories often include extracts from interviews with the midget entertainers, explaining how they enjoy what they do and thus everyone should mind their own business (Pritchard, 2023). For example, Eric Bourne, a midget entertainer who hires himself out, commented, 'I reckon people should mind their own business and if we are happy, leave us to get on with our lives' (Hall, 2019). The use of objective pronouns such as 'us' and 'we' suggests that Eric is speaking on behalf of all people with dwarfism. For centuries, midget entertainers have perpetuated a problematic representation of dwarfism which robs the rest of us of our autonomy in society. However, Watson (2020) demonstrates how representations of dwarfism are slowly changing. Aside from a few midget entertainers, people with dwarfism have been turning their backs on derogatory entertainment decades (Adelson, 2005a).

Going back to your image, perhaps you thought of Tyrion Lannister from *Game of Thrones*, played by Peter Dinklage. When offered the role it is rumoured that Dinklage demanded that there would be 'no beard, no pointy shoes' (Schulman, 2019), resisting a stereotypical portrayal of a mythical dwarf. While Dinklage's attitude has been acknowledged, the entertainment industry still promotes stereotypical depictions of dwarfism (Meeuf, 2014). To make an impact and change society's perception of dwarfism, it is important to recognise the others that are resisting and challenging the metanarrative of dwarfism. This will help to truly demonstrate to wider society that people with dwarfism are not figures of fun or mythological beings.

Voices for Change

The voices of people with dwarfism are important. Disability art is about being given a voice and about pride (Allan, 2005). As previously mentioned, representations of dwarfism have been constructed by average height people, who deem them subhuman. However, people with dwarfism are starting to challenge these representations and take back control of their autonomy. Therefore, this book gives artists and activists with dwarfism a voice to aid in promoting a more positive identity, which challenges long-held beliefs about dwarfism.

This book brings together a collective voice, which seems missing due to the fractured nature of the advocacy within the dwarfism community. There exist numerous associations for people with dwarfism around the world, including, but not limited to: The Danish Dwarf Association, Little People of America (LPA), Little People of Canada, Little People of Ireland, Little People of New Zealand and Short Statured People of Australia (SSPA). In the United Kingdom alone, there are several associations for people with dwarfism. These include the Dwarfs Sports Association UK (DSAUK), Little People UK (LPUK), Restricted Growth Association (RGA), Short Statured Scotland (SSS) and Walking with Giants. Despite the numerous associations for people with dwarfism, there seems to be limited collective advocacy for people with dwarfism. As a person with dwarfism, who is part of numerous social media groups for people with dwarfism and advocates for equality for people with the condition, I noticed that the fight against ableist conceptions of dwarfism was lacking. There are numerous reasons for this, too many to cover in this introduction. Still, one is that we are often challenged or silenced when attempting to speak out against derogatory forms of entertainment, such as midget tossing and midget wrestling (see Pritchard, 2023). However, as Branfield (1998, p. 144) states, 'we must, if we want to break from our past, be the initiators and designers of our liberation'. In other words, people with dwarfism cannot just wait for change; instead, they must be the voice to fight against derogatory representations of their condition, as opposed to the enablers. It is hoped that this book will encourage people with dwarfism and their allies to become advocates alongside those who already are.

Each chapter is written by or is based on an interview with a person with dwarfism to provide a raw and less nuanced narrative. As the editor, although I have dwarfism, I have tried to have minimal input. I felt that to provide a true voice and empowerment, the chapters needed to be written by people with dwarfism who could share their first-hand experiences of working in the arts and media. However, for numerous reasons, such as time constraints, some contributors were unable to write their own chapters. Instead, I conducted semi-structured interviews with them, and thus, my contribution is noted as 'with' them. After conducting the interview, I edited it and used it as a basis for the chapter. I expanded on parts of their interviews, often with previous research in Disability studies. I also added pseudonyms and removed names of people or organisations where relevant. The chapter was then sent back to the contributor to ensure that I had correctly interpreted their views and experiences.

When interviewing participants, my role was not to dispute their beliefs but rather to get them to expand on them. Authors were encouraged to reflect on the work they do and why. Chapters were sent to the contributors to edit, which included expanding on points and removing anything they no longer wished to include. Each chapter demonstrates that people with dwarfism do not have to abide by ableist stereotypes to work in the arts, i.e. derogatory entertainment which is often framed as 'a job for them' (Pritchard, 2023). It is often implied that actors with non-normative bodies, such as people with dwarfism, should somehow be grateful for roles that are reflective of the freak show discourse (Tyrrell, 2020). The authors offer their thoughts, experiences and importantly recommendations to improve representations of dwarfism and counteract ableist attitudes.

Throughout the book, terms such as dwarf, person with dwarfism and person of short stature appear, as authors have various reasons for adopting specific terms, based on their own sociocultural experiences of dwarfism. There are many terms used to describe someone with dwarfism, including, but not limited to: person with dwarfism, person of short stature, dwarf, little person and person of restricted growth. Most people with dwarfism accept any of these terms, although this can depend on where you are in the world. For example, little person is favoured in the United States; however, it can be met with hostility in the United Kingdom as this term is also used to refer to children. This is problematic for people with dwarfism as other people often infantilise them. Sometimes, the term 'dwarf' is also deemed distasteful by people with dwarfism, due to its connection to particular representations, including within fantasy stories and films. It can be hard to agree on an acceptable term, especially when terms associated with being small are deemed negative (Pritchard, 2023). One term the majority of people with dwarfism detest is 'midget'; however, in this book, some contributors are drawing on the concept of midgetism (see Pritchard, 2023) and reclaiming the word. Thus, in some cases, contributors refer to people with dwarfism who engage in derogatory entertainment as 'midget entertainers'. This is not an acceptance of the word midget to describe a person with dwarfism but rather as action and form of representation.

Outline of the Book

Reading and editing the following chapters and accompanying biographies have filled me with immense pride in dwarfism. I hope that others, especially those with dwarfism, who read the book also feel the same. For anyone who may not be familiar with dwarfism, I hope that you recognise that dwarfism is not a novelty but a condition that is disabling in a society made for the average-sized person. However, people with dwarfism are still capable of success. The next time a newspaper or events manager claims that midget entertainment is somehow a job for people with dwarfism, think of the people in this book. The authors come from various backgrounds, some are from a single parent household and most of them, including myself, have experienced both education and employment discrimination. Thus, if midget entertainment was our only option, this book would not exist.

The book opens with Amanda Cachia, a crip curator of artists and outspoken advocate for contemporary disability art, examining key exhibitions throughout her curating career that chart an evolution of her work towards the disability justice movement. This chapter shows how Cachia has been deploying access in her curatorial practice since 2011 intending to transform reductive interpretations of the disabled body. This chapter offers ways in which disabled people can use the arts to curate their own experiences.

Moving on, but still firmly using art as a medium for change, Debra Keenahan introduces the reader to her work as a sculptor. She argues that to adequately represent her embodied experience through her art requires the representation of the dynamic subjective process of identity formation. Through the sculptural encounter, Keenahan's intention is for viewers to experience the corporeal, spatial and relational dynamics which communicate that a person with dwarfism is an 'Other'. Whereas Keenahan wants to engage viewers not as if they are engaging with her, but rather as if the sculpture is engaging with the viewer as if the viewer is her. That is, Keenahan endeavours to achieve the dynamic of reverse audiencing of the female dwarf through the oppositional gaze.

While the first two chapters demonstrate the importance of art, in Chapter 3, *Where are the Creative Opportunities for People with Dwarfism Lived Experience in Participatory Arts Funding?* Steph Robson argues that there is an urgent need for institutional support, time, funding, development, research and mentorship in creative opportunities for the dwarfism community. She proposes how this can be achieved, primarily through participatory arts, whether as professionals, individuals or as groups. This chapter opens up more forms of engagement with art but demonstrates how there is often a lack of support which can hinder people's engagement with art as a form of advocacy.

The book then moves on to how performers with dwarfism refuse to engage in roles that reinforce stereotypes. In Chapter 4, Alice Lambert, performance artist and actor, takes the reader through her journey in becoming a performer whose work pushes for equality. In the first part, we discuss how she became a performer. While she will openly tell anyone who asks, 'Yes, I have done Snow White and the Seven Dwarfs', in this chapter, Lambert unpicks her experience and gives an explanation so that people can understand why she would never do that role ever again. She reflects on how it was promoted as a positive form of employment for people with dwarfism and how activists were constructed negatively by those in the industry. Through time, hard work and perseverance, Alice explains how the narrative which runs through her work has always got some acknowledgement of dwarfism and equal rights.

In Chapter 5, Tamm Reynolds, aka Midgitte Bardot, reflects upon how engaging in drag performances allows them to push for a more positive and realistic dwarf identity through political performances. Reynolds, who can be considered a crip, queer solo performer, believes that having a drag alter ego permits them to do anything with an air of confidence that someone like them is usually not afforded. In this case, it is to be sexy, while exposing the everyday discrimination they face as a person with dwarfism. Referring to herself as a 'political freak', Reynolds demonstrates how she engages in shock performance to raise awareness. In particular, within this chapter, Reynolds includes a poem she recites to audiences to express the psycho-emotional disablism she faces as a result of the actions of one performer who often engages in midget entertainment (Pritchard, 2023).

In Chapter 6, Danny Woodburn, acclaimed actor and disability activist, details how throughout his career he has had to negotiate with writers and producers who have often resorted to engaging with problematic stereotypes of dwarfism in their productions. While Woodburn has an admirable career and starred in many films and television shows, most notably Seinfeld, this chapter demonstrates how his success has not been easy. As a result, Woodburn discusses his role as an activist in the industry, including how he confronts the controversial practice of cripping up through what he terms the Woodburn ratio. This chapter provides an insight into how the film industry is often inaccessible for disabled actors, which can limit opportunities.

In Chapter 7, Simon Minty, founder of Abnormally Funny People and Board Member of the National Theatre, explores the successes and the not-so-positive moments of his career. Keeping with the theme of positive representations, Minty shows how the depictions of people with dwarfism have shifted to start to include more realistic representation and how this can impact an individual's confidence, identity and they are treated. Minty also demonstrates how challenging these depictions can lead to more interesting and creative work.

Further developing the push for more positive representations of dwarfism, in Chapter 8, Nic Novicki, creator of Easterseals Disability Film Challenge, reflects on his career as an actor, writer and producer with dwarfism. Novicki explains how he was able to get work for himself by creating his own projects, which opened up the door for him to play roles that were not defined by his height. As a result, Novicki discusses how he was inspired to create opportunities for other disabled people, including actors and creators with dwarfism, through the creation of the Easterseals Disability Film Challenge – a film-making competition where each film must include a disabled person. Novicki argues that taking your career in your own hands opens up the door for telling authentic stories, and it also leads to opportunities for better representations of dwarfism. This also enables what Nic terms 'dwarf pride', pride that we should have in ourselves as people with dwarfism.

Moving on from performers, the next set of chapters focuses on how other people with dwarfism advocate using different platforms. In Chapter 9 *Dwarfism Advocacy: A Lifetime Appointment [Or] A Life Tenure*, Angela Muir van Etten, lawyer and former president of LPA, gives readers a thorough insight into her life as an activist. In this chapter, van Etten provides a review of how to advocate against negative encounters with the public and is presented with the underlying premise that dwarfs should be accepted as equal contributing members of society. A discussion of systems advocacy against dwarf tossing and environmental barriers is presented within a framework of effective advocacy principles that can be applied to any situation. Van Etten shows that advocacy makes change possible when people care enough to do something, commit to the cause for as long as it takes, collaborate and form coalitions with like-minded people and communicate with honesty and respect.

In Chapter 10, Kara B Ayers reflects on her evolution as both a content creator with dwarfism and a researcher who studies disability portrayals in the media. Ayers specifically explores her intentionality to share glimpses into her life as a mother with dwarfism and a disability advocate. While we need more representations of dwarfism in the media overall, Ayers argues for the priority of quality over quantity given the pitfalls of inspiration porn and similar objectifying portrayals. Ayers offers some recommendations for a more positive representation of dwarfism on social media.

Continuing with how media can be used to challenge misconceptions about dwarfism; Jillian Curwin, founder and owner of the podcast *Always Looking Up*, reflects on her work as a podcast host. She argues that podcasts have become a platform to amplify voices that are not often heard in mainstream media on a wide range of topics. In Chapter 11, Curwin demonstrates how she has used this platform to create and to raise awareness on issues affecting the dwarfism and disabled communities. Specifically, Curwin discusses how the conversations she has had, including with prominent activists within the disability community, have resonated with listeners across the globe. Curwin argues that a podcast episode creates a space for ideas for change to be shared and lessons to be learned. As a result, she argues that organisations such as Little People of America should have their own podcast to inform, educate and advocate because people are listening.

In Chapter 12, Sam Drummond details how he found his 'voice' both on the radio and through writing his memoir *Broke*. Drummond provides readers with an insight into his life as a man with dwarfism, from a single parent family, demonstrating how memoir can be used to showcase the intersectional life of someone with dwarfism. Drummond describes how problematic representations have impacted social encounters throughout his life, which are presented within his memoir. This chapter shows another way for people with dwarfism to challenge problematic representations by showing their real-life impact.

In the last chapter, Emily Sullivan-Sanford presents her experience with limb-lengthening, addressing the enormous social pressure to be normal in appearance, illustrating this pressure with personal, anecdotal and statistical evidence. Height altering treatments are a controversial topic within the dwarfism community. I felt it was important to include the voice of a person with dwarfism who has had limb-lengthening surgery. Sullivan-Sanford recommends that both realistic and idealistic representations of people with dwarfism are required in mainstream media. These goals are the basis of her work with online platforms and the diversity workshops that she leads. This last chapter helps the reader to consider some of the arguments in the previous chapters and how they are constructed by ableist ideas inherent within society.

References

Adelson, B. (2005a). The changing lives of archetypal 'curiosities' – And echoes of the past. *Disability Studies Quarterly*, *25*(3), 1–13.

Adelson, B. (2005b). *The lives of dwarfs: Their journey from public curiosity toward social liberation*. Rutgers University Press.

Allan, J. (2005). Encounters with exclusion through disability arts. *Journal of Research in Special Educational Needs, 5*(1), 31–36.

Bolt, D. (2019). *Cultural disability studies in education*. Routledge.

Bolt, D. (Ed.). (2021). *The metanarrative of disability: Culture, assumed authority, and the normative social order*. Routledge.

Branfield, F. (1998). What are you doing here? 'Non-disabled' people and the disability movement: A response to Robert F. Drake. *Disability & Society, 13*(1), 143–144.

Ellis, L. (2018). Through a filtered lens: Unauthorized picture taking of people with dwarfism in public spaces. *Disability & Society, 33*(2), 218–237.

Haberer, J. (2010). *The little difference: dwarfism and the media*. Norderstedt.

Hall, D. (2019). Baby shambles expectant mums paying dwarfs £300 to dress up as newborns for baby showers. *The Sun* [online]. https://www.thesun.co.uk/news/8520698/mums-hiring-300-dwarfs-for-baby-showers/. Accessed on February 04, 2024.

Meeuf, R. (2014). The nonnormative celebrity body and the meritocracy of the star system: Constructing Peter Dinklage in entertainment journalism. *Journal of Communication Inquiry, 38*(3), 204–222.

Mock, S. (2020). "Against a dwarf": The medieval motif of the antagonistic dwarf and its role in contemporary literature and film. *Journal of Literary & Cultural Disability Studies, 14*(2), 155–170.

Pritchard, E. (2021). The metanarrative of dwarfism: Heightism and its social implications. In D. Bolt (Ed.), *The metanarrative of disability: Culture, assumed authority, and the normative social order* (pp. 123–137). Routledge.

Pritchard, E. (2023). *Midgetism: The exploitation and discrimination of people with dwarfism*. Routledge.

Pritchard, E., & Kruse, R. (2020). Introduction: Cultural representations of dwarfism. *Journal of Literary & Cultural Disability Studies, 14*(2), 131–135.

Schulman, M. (2019). Peter Dinklage is still punk rock. *The New Yorker* [online]. https://www.newyorker.com/culture/the-new-yorker-interview/peter-dinklage-is-still-punk-rock. Accessed on July 23, 2023.

Tan, N. C. (2021). "Thrilla in Manila": Troubling theatricality and uneasy spectator affects surrounding the ringside bar midget boxing and wrestling. *The Asian Journal of Literature, Culture, Performance, 1*(2), 1–13.

Tyrrell, B. (2020). A world turned upside down: Hip-frog, freak shows, and representations of dwarfism. *Journal of Literary & Cultural Disability Studies, 14*(2), 171–186.

Watson, K. (2020). "With and smile and a song": Representations of people with dwarfism in 1930s cinema. *Journal of Literary & Cultural Disability Studies, 14*(2), 137–153.

Chapter 1

Curating New Perspectives: How My Dwarfism Led Me to Disability Art

Amanda Cachia (Professor, Curator and Writer)

USA

My place as a curator and writer in the art world is that I have personal experience with scale and size norms. I have a rare form of dwarfism called brachyolmia – and I'm 4'3" (129 cm) tall (Mayo Clinic, 2023). I am using the word 'dwarf' in this essay as I refer to myself as a person with dwarfism, as these are the terms I have always used to identify myself as. I have faster bone degeneration than the ostensible average-height person, spinal stenosis and scoliosis. While I have never had to have any surgery as an outcome of my dwarfism, I have had to deal with the social and cultural stigma attached to having a body that is considered atypical and startlingly noticeable in the public eye. As a consequence, I often have to negotiate the challenges of staring, occasional comments and questions and living in a world that has been architecturally designed for the so-called 'average' six-foot person (Biggers, 2019). What one might see as a physical difference – my short stature – that becomes a disability when not accommodated in a world of normative-scaled design is also critically sensory with respect to gaze and access. This chapter will examine key exhibitions throughout my curating career that chart an evolution of my work towards the disability justice movement.

I began this work by first thinking about artists who had the same conditions as myself. I had met Irish artist Corban Walker at my first Little People of America convention back in 2005 in Minneapolis, and then I saw him again at the opening of his exhibition representing the Irish Pavilion at the Venice Biennale in 2011. I flew to Venice from Oakland, California (where I was living at the time), specifically to see Walker in Venice, at one of the world's most prestigious art events. I knew I could not miss this opportunity to witness a person with achondroplasia taking centre stage in this highly prestigious professional art world context. It was Walker's work that made its way into my first disability-themed exhibition in 2012 at the Cantor Fitzgerald Gallery at Haverford College in Pennsylvania, entitled *What Can a Body Do?* which was inspired by French philosopher Gilles Deleuze's thinking as he grappled with Spinoza's

---

Dwarfism Arts and Advocacy, 11–23
Copyright © 2024 Amanda Cachia
Published under exclusive licence by Emerald Publishing Limited
doi:10.1108/978-1-83753-922-220241003

question, 'What can a body do?' or, in my exhibition's underlying specificity, 'What can a *disabled* body do?'

While Walker has made representational work exploring his literal embodiment, he is mostly interested in making sculptural installations that rely on minimalist cues and traditions. I found Walker's work to be the most compelling of the small handful of artists with dwarfism I had discovered during my research, both because of his steer away from the representational, but also because it was a powerful entry point to the sensory. He is, in fact, the only artist with dwarfism I'm aware of who is not interested in the politics of representation, which is why I found him to be so refreshing. I remember being very intrigued about his work, as I simultaneously struggled to understand it – I asked myself, what can we learn about the disabled body in art when no disabled body is physically present? Walker found a compelling way to do this through sensorial and phenomenological channels, and, as I discovered in the years after our first meeting, so did other disabled artists. I had unlocked a key to a new world of understanding embodiment, albeit through the stigmatised lens of the now-abstract disabled corpus. However, I also recognised that perhaps these new methodologies for understanding embodiment were a gateway in which to challenge reductive assumptions.

Indeed, spatial experiences of dwarfism, like other disabilities, offer a subjugated knowledge and a way of thinking about aesthetics differently. As a person with a rare form of dwarfism, it was important to me to see how my body (and those of other disabled artists) might find space in the museum or in the discourse of art history textbooks. When I was a graduate student at the California College of the Arts in San Francisco, and writing my master's thesis on Corban Walker and Laura Swanson (another artist with achondroplasia), I decided to build my own custom-sized lectern which I dubbed *Alterpodium* in collaboration with furniture design students for the purpose of delivering my thesis presentation in the college's large auditorium. I made this environment work for me, instead of having to adjust to the literal misfit of the predetermined built space around me. This seemed like a good way to enact and empower the spatial and phenomenological experiences I had on a daily basis, and to take more complex roles as an activist, designer, performer and scholar. In the paragraphs to follow, I share how my height has been implicated in my job as a curator, followed by a deeper discussion on how the work of Corban Walker challenges means of moving and displaying art in the museum from the dwarf perspective. I then pair this with a discussion on several case studies of exhibitions I have curated in the past decade that also set up antagonistic and challenging strategies for moving through the gallery space for non-disabled audiences to raise awareness of dwarf and disabled embodiment.

How to Hang Like an Ableist Curator

Back in 2002, I held my first job as a full-time institutional curator at the New England Regional Art Museum in Armidale, New South Wales, Australia, which required me to learn the ropes of installing art exhibitions. I did everything from leading a troop of reliable volunteers who would hang multiple rooms of art on the walls to climbing up scaffolds and adjusting the spotlights on the tall ceiling tracks, to cutting up foam core with a sharp blade to create labels. As the curator, I would also make artwork selections, liaise with artists to develop biographical and interpretive text and install the vinyl signage on the walls. I would also be the bearer of bad news for artists when their artwork would occasionally get damaged during shipment (which means the gallery did not bear responsibility). The work of hanging the art on the walls was the most labour-intensive. This particular gallery did not want to drill holes into the walls which would require constant patch-up and paint work after the shows came down, so they had a permanent mini-rail system installed along the top section of all their ten-foot-high walls. Attached to the rail were hooks and cords, and the art would then hang off the cords using the two D-rings screwed to the back of the left and right side of the artwork frame. I remember being taught how to hang the work, and it would begin by using expandable reacher poles to fasten the hook and cord to the rail along the top of the wall – quite a task in itself. Then, I was taught how to determine the spacing of the works along the length of the wall, by subtracting the length of the overall wall with the length of the works, so that the works were evenly divided up for equal spacing. I was taught to hang the work at eye level, and we used 60″ (152 cm) as the measurement for the centre point of hanging the work, which would be marked on the wall with a pencil or with blue painter's tape. I was also taught how to engage in this measuring process using a red laser. Once the work was attached to the cords using the D-rings, we would use a level to ensure the work was straight, and then the finishing piece was to adjust the spotlight over the work for the optimum viewing experience. While not every gallery or museum uses the mini-rail system with cords to affix their artworks to the wall, the procedure I was taught was very much 'standard' or 'typical'.

Now that I was privy to the machinations of display, I was let into a world that most visitors are unaware of when they look at a work of art, and indeed, why should they? Hang-height, for example, is quite meaningless when it compliments their body type. But the presumed comfort of 60″ hang-height is not everyone's experience and is not seemingly 'natural' for everyone. In fact, from another perspective, it's a socially exclusionary mechanism whose power to divide society rests on many museum visitors simply taking this for granted. As a person and a curator with dwarfism at 4′3″ (129 cm) tall, my experience viewing exhibitions in galleries and museums is characterised by quite a different spatial orientation. I look upwards towards works of art hung on the wall. The 'standard' height is too high for me to adequately see it, mirroring my embodied intersubjective exchange with other average-height bodies. By this, I mean that when I am in conversation with 'leggies' (a colloquial term that my husband, who also has achondroplasia, uses to describe people of average height), I am also looking up at them. In tandem with this challenging experience of looking at objects high up on walls is how I am also 'blinded' by certain spatial and physical conditions in my greater environment, along with how I am occasionally 'deafened' as well. For example, given that audio components are sometimes embedded into a work of art that is also hung at this standard height, out of ear's reach for my stature, this means that I cannot hear it as well as not be able to see it. This formula also applies to my intersubjective relationship to other human bodies, given that the sound to emanate from a voice that is much taller than me is often lost on my ears, particularly when I am ensconced in a noisy environment, such as a gallery opening, which makes hearing even more difficult.

Of course, to compound the apparent unthinkable naturalness of hang-height for the viewing experience is the fact that as a young curator, I was trained by experienced average-height museum professionals to install art in this way, despite their being aware of my very visible short stature. Hang-height was never questioned, nor was it ever discussed regarding how the museum might use me as a new resource or barometer in which to challenge conventions and consider new possibilities for different types and sizes of bodies that might walk or roll through the museum's doors and engage with art. It makes me both sad and angry that the needs of my body were rendered invisible and unimportant by my colleagues – not on purpose certainly but simply because standards are entrenched and considered normal, while my body was the piece of the puzzle that fell literally out of the line of vision.

One time, at the beginning of my career, during a job interview for a curatorial position, I was asked how I was going to hang the art given that installing exhibitions was one of the job responsibilities. The interviewer assumed this would be difficult for me and seemed concerned that I was not going to be able to literally meet the criteria owing to my short stature. I responded that I would simply use ladders and step stools, and I used a tone of voice that indicated it was not an issue of concern, but the interviewer did not look convinced. I did not get the job. Clearly, the issue of hang-height and any possible deviation to the standard did not cross the interviewer's mind; I was the one that did not measure up, both to the spot on the wall where works had to be hung and, ultimately and frustratingly, to the job itself. I regret that I have perpetuated this same hang-height museum standard in many exhibitions I have curated over the past 20 years across many gallery spaces because of the difficulty of being a lone dissenter in the mainstream and the fear of speaking out. More frankly, I also feared coming out as disabled. But eventually, I knew it was time to change, and that I needed to speak up.

In 2014, I curated *Composing Dwarfism* at Space4Art in San Diego during the Little People of America convention, which included the work of Ricardo Gil and Laura Swanson. I wanted to provide an activist space in which little people in my community could see photographs of themselves taken by themselves, rather than through narrow and limited tropes of the sensationalistic nude dwarf or the dwarf as entertainer as commonly depicted through modernist photographers such as Diane Arbus or Arthur Fellig and other earlier periods in art history. It was a successful display, but what I found to be more important and pressing, of course, than the representations of generative dwarf embodiment in the photographs was the height at which the works of art were hung. I purposefully hung the work much lower on the gallery wall, to suit the needs of a person with dwarfism, who is on average four feet. I used 4ft (120 cm) as the measurement for the centre point of the work instead of 60″ (152 cm). This remains a spatial orientation and phenomenological experience that needs to be urgently and consistently addressed in museum and gallery practice. In the next section, I discuss how the work of Corban Walker has begun to address the unique spatial and phenomenological orientation of dwarfism in the museum.

Disrupting Mobility and Vision

Upon entering the gallery, the viewer sees several rows of stainless-steel wire cable lines strung from one side of the gallery wall to the other, suspended approximately four feet above the ground. Then, upon walking to another section of the gallery, the lines begin again and repeat themselves, threading from one side of the room to the next, again using the dimension of four feet as an elevation point from the ground, up to the lowest row of the steel lines. As the name implies, *Trapezoid* (1997), the artist is attempting to trap or ensnare the visitor into this throng of lines, disrupting one's smooth pathway so that one is forced to consider an alternative through bending, crouching, twisting or turning to get to the other side of the lines and to the other side of the gallery. As a man with achondroplasia, the most common form of dwarfism, Corban Walker uses his height as a measuring point for the elevation of the lines, so that he disrupts the average-height viewer's spatial flow as they walk through a gallery space. Walker claims spatial agency in a domain that usually privileges the average-height viewing position, where paintings are hung at a so-called universal and standard eye level.

Walker's work often relates to architectural scale and spatial perception, utilising industrial materials such as steel, aluminium and glass, drawing on minimalism to highlight different perspectives in relation to height and scale. As someone who is four feet tall (120 cm), he creates his sculpture stacks in direct proportion to his body using the 'Corban rule', a precise mathematical calculation he devised, wherein he uses his own height as a measure of his art. This spurs viewers to think about the built environment in different terms. Walker has talked about how he tries to get viewers to move as they encounter his works from new positions. The starting point for Walker's praxis is the dimensions of his physical stature, which 'he multiplies and morphs [into] the dimensions of his works to make manifest the normally invisible systems that govern our movements' (Hanson, 2011). Walker provides a point of view that refuses the typical, normal or average. For audiences of average-height, bending down to see the installation shifts 'standard-sized' audiences from their usual, un-thought-about looking straight-on viewpoint of an artwork. Walker wants to focus on drawing people downwards, closer to the ground, into a dimension equivalent to the 'Corban scale'. Given Walker's height of four feet, he usually has to crane his neck to look up at people's faces or reach up to shake someone's hand in his everyday reality. *Trapezoid* reverses this 'staturization of space' (which means 'the dominant preference for able bodies of an average height') (Kruse, 2010).

The Corban rule adds a fascinating and evocative intervention and juxtaposition with other human scale devices, such as Leonardo da Vinci's *Vitruvian Man* (1487) and Le Corbusier's *Modulor* (1943). The *Modulor*, in particular, is an anthropometric scale of proportions devised by the Swiss-born French architect. It is based on the six-foot height of an Englishman with his arm raised. These measurements do not represent the diversity, form and shape of all bodies, and these measurements translated into architecture and our built environment create barriers for disabled people. The iconic image of *Vitruvian Man* incorporates a perfect concentric circle in a thinly drawn line that represents the cyclical and uninterrupted flow of so-called 'normal' up and down movement that the arms should make at the side of the body; the legs are engaged in similar gestures back and forth, but it especially demonstrates proportion and symmetry, and that a body in proportion and with symmetry is a body that fits within a pristine circle. These art historical aesthetic ideals of perfection, proportion and beauty are found in classical sculpture and modernism and in architecture through the golden section. The golden section is an average measure conforming to man. Regretfully, the widespread representation of a bodily ideal in *Vitruvian Man* and *Modulor* in art history contributes to ableist attitudes and discrimination against the disabled minority. This is because there is an internalised, almost unconscious assumption of able-bodiedness in art theory and praxis – if the assumption becomes 'disrupted' by non-normative corporeal forms, then these forms have historically been rejected and marked as pathological, diseased and 'other'. While bodily ideals have shifted in art (such as the mannerist bodies of the late 16th century or rococo bodies), the primary narrative of art history still goes back to the Da Vinci/Corbusier norm, and they remain especially dominant in popular culture.

Corban Walker's own Corban rule works as an antithesis to these deeply entrenched ideals, echoing a broader tradition of installations that force audience members to change their experience of space, ranging from Marcel Duchamp to Bruce Nauman. Through Walker's lines of string or stainless steel, the ideal of the framed painting is also negated as there are now additional conceptual and multi-modal layers to consider. The viewer is forced to reflect on the physical context and their own participation in the production or experience of any meaning in the encounter with art objects. This is the axis in which the work of Walker spins, as his work provides embodied encounters to the public that act to reveal the artificial construction of conventional gallery spaces and 'normal' viewing experiences. Here, the sensorium of disability renders alternative meanings that make explicit and expressive the often hidden inter-relationships between body size, art object and movements through space.

Walker's antagonistic work, which has consistently aimed to manipulate and disrupt movement, can be seen in more recent installations, although this time, with more gravitational pull, literally. In the fall of 2015, Walker completed a residency at Atelier Calder in France. During his time there, he completed a new work entitled *Short Minute Matter*, which consists of 88 painted steel stanchions which he both found and made, and then connected them with a long and winding stainless steel cable. In this work, the artist is once again manipulating the typical and straight-forward navigational pathway for a gallery and museum visitor as they engage with a work of art, as this installation is set up to mimic a labyrinth of sorts. As one traverses through the rows of stanchions and lines of cable framing the path, one must determine how to get out of the installation shortly upon entering. Walker has created this installation as a response to his personal experience with stanchions and cables when engaging with works of art in museums in Europe. Stanchions are typically a tool that museums use as a way to ensure that visitors do not get too close to a valuable painting or sculpture, and of course they are also meant to ward off any temptations to touch a work, which is also forbidden. Stanchions are often installed alongside alarms, which go off if a visitor's shins graze the cable, indicating they have gotten too close and therefore issuing a caution to avoid such close contact. In Walker's own experience, stanchions, while certainly warding him off from getting too close, also happen to greet his body at a higher point on his body owing to his short stature, and they become quite a nuisance and quite an extraordinary interruption to his artwork viewing. *Short Minute Matter*, then, has unfolded as a response to Walker's irritation and frustration with getting tangled up in stanchions. The word 'matter' in the title of the work alludes to both the matter of the steel from which they're made, but of course it also references the 'issue' at hand. This is a matter that takes a short minute to untangle from, as Walker's short body gets tripped up on its unwelcoming fence line. Walker's stanchions are aimed to be intentionally interrupting of a visitor's spatial orientation through the Calder exhibition space, but he also wants to point out the fact of stanchions and their unfavourable qualities to begin with. I imagine that average-height viewers may experience mild annoyance with stanchions when visiting famous works of art in museums, but in Walker's installation, one's encounter with stanchions becomes magnified because one cannot avoid them and cannot help but be entangled in them owing to the nature of Walker's labyrinthine concoction. Walker states, 'you have to navigate through the labyrinth to find your way out without tripping over the stanchions, which are nicely glowing in the sunlight [as if taunting you to engage and get twisted up]' (Walker, 2022). He wants the average-height viewer to experience some of the frustration that he experiences on a regular basis during his own interrupted viewing experience of art, and I imagine he is quite successful with his imperative.

Curating and Disrupting Movement

In this section, I discuss three different exhibitions I have curated in the past decade that demonstrate how I have also set up antagonistic and challenging strategies for moving through the gallery space for non-disabled audiences to raise awareness of dwarf and disabled embodiment. In *Performing Crip Time*, held at Space4Art gallery in downtown San Diego in 2014, I installed a video installation of an outdoor performance by British artist Noëmi Laikmaer. In the documentation of the living intervention/performance, *One Morning in May* (2012), on the 28th of May, Lakmaier set out from Toynbee Studios in Tower Hamlets towards the City of London, hoping to reach one of London's most iconic buildings, the 'Gherkin'. Lakmaier has made a choice to discard and abandon her wheelchair temporarily, while she circulates and sometimes rolls her body in and around a familiar route of London on hands and knees, and occasionally stops for breaks to rest her deteriorating body and observe bustling city life. This normally easy one mile stroll was a slow and exhausting test of endurance. Smartly dressed in business attire, she crawled through the everyday street life of London, her clothes getting increasingly dirty and torn. After 7 hours, she crossed the border from the Borough of Tower Hamlets to the City of London, and at the end of her arduous journey, her business suit now torn and soiled from the grime of the city's worn streets, she smokes a cigarette to commemorate its conclusion.

The video was presented on a flat screen television which I decided to install on the concrete floor of the gallery, rather than mounting it to the wall or propping it up on a waist-high pedestal for more comfortable viewing for average-height visitors. I enjoyed making an aesthetic conceptual connection between Noëmi as she crawled across the concrete pavements of London in comparison with the flat screen placed on the floors of the gallery. The effect gave a powerful illusion, and it was almost as if Noëmi was crawling on the very floors of the gallery itself. However, my curatorial intervention was much more than creative access in this instance. Similar to the antagonistic ways that many contemporary disabled artists, including Corban Walker, have engaged with their audience as a primary methodology, so too did I have a more antagonistic curatorial approach towards the audience, as the average-height visitor was going to be somewhat uncomfortable in their efforts to watch the work, by either hunching down, bending or crouching to see the work on the floor. Given my shorter stature, it was far easier for me to see it, or anyone in a wheelchair, than for someone of average height, thus I was considering and favouring certain disabled embodiments first in the execution of this installation.

The Flesh of the World was a 24-person exhibition that I curated in summer 2015 across three different gallery spaces at the University of Toronto. Inspired by the 2015 XVII Pan American and Parapan American Games and the work of Merleau-Ponty, *The Flesh of the World* was an exhibition presenting diverse and complex views of the body that might deepen qualities typically associated with competitive sports and games, such as the relationship between the body and technology, and how the senses might offer new forms of knowledge to corporeal performance and potential. *The Flesh of the World* pushed the limits of the body and challenged dominant culture's understanding of normativity and embodiment through work by Canadian and international artists who use the body as a medium. The artists critically inquired and experimented with the shape and forms of bodies, proving that, within the context of both the exhibition and the field of athleticism itself, the body is unfixed and indeterminate. The exhibition also made important connections between the language of complex embodiment and the language of sports, given that many of the issues relating to endurance, physical limits, failure, pathos and the human psyche inform both these fields. It is within the confluence of these two worlds, sometimes playful, sometimes reflective, that we can radically expand our ideas of the corporeal apparatus as a whole.

The works spanned across various media, including film and video installation, sculptures, framed photographs, drawings, paintings and several performances. The exhibition aimed to emphasise how visitors might engage with this work across multidisciplinary, multi-modal platforms. Just like the Pan Am and Parapan Am Games itself, this project offered up the artists' work to the audience through a wider fulcrum of knowing the contours of our flesh.

Contemporary exhibitions that touch on disability-related themes and subject matter often fall into two common interpretations: one that reductively and simplistically equates the person (usually the artist) with their disability and the other that regards disability as an index of our shared humanness. In *The Flesh of the World*, I aimed to offer this nuanced approach to issues of complex embodiment. The exhibition aimed to suggest that there is no one monolithic definition of disability and resisted relying on an all-too-easy template or discursive framework based on the uniformity of other marginalised identity categories such as gender, race or sexuality. This was conveyed through a lack of uniformity of the bodies that were on display, and while one might perceive a possible ghettoisation of subjects based purely on their diagnostic determinations, I evaded this problem endemic to many exhibitions bringing together disability and art by not programming it exclusively with art about disability. In this show, some artists identified as disabled, while many others did not. Through a hybrid selection of works, some requiring direct visitor participation and engagement, I aimed to draw the viewer into a new understanding of 'adaptation', in the hopes that the primitive idea that disabilities must be 'overcome' can very slowly be erased. By offering an exhibition like this, where articulation of disability is often misunderstood and easily misinterpreted, the politics of complex embodiment were not only visible on a multi-modal stage, but they were performed: by the artists certainly and especially by the audience.

The exhibition contained three variations of Canadian-based artist Mowry Baden's untitled *Seatbelt* devices, *Untitled (Seat Belt, Three Points)*, 1970, *Untitled (Seat Belt with Concrete Block)*, 1969–1970, and *Untitled (Seat Belt with Pole and Two Straps)*, 1969–1970, which were installed at each of the three exhibition venues across two separate campuses. This three-pronged series of physical pivotal sculptures that rotate around a centre point reflects Baden's interest in movement and its impact on perception and required that viewers interact with, and physically operate them, demonstrating the artist's performative and collaborative approach with the audience. While these works are arguably visually bland, once you strap yourself into the devices and begin to unevenly circle the central anchor point, one is able to grasp the experience of moving with a body that is not completely under your control. Through this interactive work, Baden illustrates a shared human ability to adapt to bodily circumstances that shift and alter. Indeed, through the *Untitled Seatbelt* series, Baden is unwittingly turning the viewers' attention to a notion of complex embodiment. The sense-experience of travelling in an interrupted circle while strapped into a device that modifies movement offers new knowledge. The adaptations the body makes under these new ambulatory circumstances are necessarily creative and inventive, for one must learn how to navigate space differently: physically, cognitively and multi-sensorially. One may come to appreciate newly discovered bodily skill, form, shape and gesture or revel in the choreographic possibilities under this new corporeal regime that blends together objects, bodies and space in a dynamic, evolving environment. Certainly, Baden achieves these outcomes through this work, and while the effect of the body in motion under the reins of the re-contextualised seatbelts is subtle, I argue that it also attempts to draw the viewer into an equation with the artists in the exhibition and the larger community of people with disabilities (Dick, 2015).

Through *The Flesh of the World*, I sought to disrupt the ideals of ostensible correct form, shape and movement ingrained in art history, both through audience interaction and observation at the level of horizontality. I did this by curating many works into the exhibition that had the capacity to engage the audience. During the installation and opening of the show in June 2015, I had strapped on Baden's *Untitled (Seat Belt with Concrete Block)* and walked around in disrupted concentric circles in a clockwise direction because I was raising and placing one leg repeatedly on my right side whenever my body would inevitably encounter the concrete block that seemed determined to block my path within the circular journey. I had to step and climb over the concrete block to maintain consistent movement and keep on my way. The concrete block caused my hip to rise up uncomfortably, and in the process, it served to remind me of the curvature in my spine or scoliosis. I could not tell whether the up and down movement on my right side was balancing my always already off-kilter stature, as the curvature causes one side of my body to be slightly raised and higher than the other. I thought that perhaps a tingling pain from my spinal stenosis as a result of my brachyolmia might also be triggered by the negotiation of objects in space, but it was not. After several sequences of this gesture, I stopped and undid the seat belt and returned to my own daily version of complex embodiment, distinct and yet in parallel with Baden's series given both require ambulatory adjustments of being in the world.

My experience of this work demonstrates how an empirical turn towards disability in curatorial practice and art history at large can be premised on one that *moves*, as this movement was offering new knowledge through direct physical engagement. In other words, to curate an audience moving and experimenting through adaptation is to get an audience thinking about and empathising with disability and dwarfism differently, in a bid to transform entrenched reductive attitudes.

Asking the audience to 'move' within an installation is a way of bringing the audience into a zone of engagement with the disabled subject, therefore emphasising that a new model of reception and experience would be catalysed in this relationship between the viewer and the *non-normative* body. In their acts of physically moving, the participant/viewer is effectively and compassionately moved as well. As I have already shown, there are many examples that demonstrate how this 'movement' is enacted by the artists (the non-disabled or disabled subject, as the case may be), and as a consequence, how these physical gestures may impact the audience member, either through direct participation, or by viewership, which I argue is in itself, a type of sense that carries particular politics.

Through this participatory movement, the audience member is motivated to 'be with' the disabled subject, and to also, hopefully, shed their reductive associations with the disabled body that may have larger consequences on instilling social changes towards the treatment of the disabled subject. Through these analyses, I demonstrate how the artists procure a new perspective from the participant and/or viewer that brings them into a shared sense of the disabled subject's vulnerability, suffering and corporal conditions. The idea is that through this participation, some semblance of the disabled subject's various complex embodiments will bridge any gap or distance between the so-called 'able' and the 'disabled' and instead demonstrate a shared humanity in which we all partake, differently.

In *Automatisme Ambulatoire: Hysteria, Imitation, Performance*, which I curated for the Owens Art Gallery at Mt. Saint Allison University in Sackville, New Brunswick in 2019, I commissioned six artists to develop new works focused on choreography and installation through ideas of 'automatisme ambulatoire', 'hysteria' and 'epilepsy' as a performance style. The artists also considered how these gestures can work to subvert, undo, transform and re-imagine the body and language, both real and imagined. 'Ambulatory automatism' is an expression that conjures notions of the compulsive traveller, while simultaneously implying irresistible urges and movements such as grimaces, tics and gestures that form relationships with corporeal pathologies. The exhibition took as its departure point an essay by scholar Rae Beth Gordon, which focuses on unconscious imitation and spectatorship in French cabaret and early cinema. In Gordon's essay, she seeks to find correlation between the movement that was staged in early cinema with that of the movement of hysteria, epilepsy, catalepsy and other contractures of the body. Gordon felt that hysterical gesture and gait were 'important inspirations for the style of frenetic, anarchic movement' that was present in early French film comedy, which had as its predecessor a clear inspiration of nervous pathology in cabaret and concert performances, both on and off the screen.[1] Indeed, Gordon suggests that these shaking, convulsing, agitating movements of the lower order of the body symbolised the body taking over reason and thus led towards an essential loss of control. It is this pathological notion of loss of control, popular during the 18th and 19th centuries, which Gordon surmised came to be almost synonymous with 'modernity' itself. Artists and poets, in addition to cabaret performers, actors and film-makers, all came to be deeply influenced by 'hysteria'. Surrealist artist Andre Breton described it this way: 'Hysteria is a mental state...characterised by the subversion of the relationships established between the subject and the moral world...it can, from every point of view, be considered as a supreme means of expression'.[2] Through their diverse and established choreographic practices, which always already embrace hybrid performance-based gestures, these artists aimed to question, challenge and

---

[1] Rae Beth Gordon, 'From Charcot to Charlot: Unconscious Imitation and Spectatorship in French Cabaret and Early Cinema', in *The Mind of Modernism: Medicine, Psychology, and the Cultural Arts in Europe and America, 1880–1940*, Mark S. Micale (ed.), Stanford, California: Stanford University Press, 2004, 94.
[2] Breton quoted by Gordon, Ibid., 124.

complicate the ethical and moral boundaries of 'imitation', and how the so-called 'pathologised' body might be considered under new social and cultural contemporary contexts. Through their work, they charted an evolution of the moving corpus since modern times. Through this exhibition, I argued that it is especially through the performance and portrayal of queer, disabled and gendered subjects that the ambulatory hysteric could be reclaimed, rethought and revitalised within a social justice context.

One of the major installations in this exhibition that captured my thematic brilliantly was by Scottish choreographer and performer Claire Cunningham. *Tributary* (2019) toured to Sackville, New Brunswick, after having already been presented theatrically across a number of venues in the United Kingdom just prior to its debut in Canada. *Tributary* explored ideas of impersonation and tribute by Elvis Presley tribute artists and links them to the ways disabled individuals may have been conditioned through medical interventions from childhood to strive for some mythical or iconic body. Looking through and into the world of the professional tribute artist, Cunningham's work also examined notions of the spectacle and control, as well as the provocation of disturbing bodies and the re-appropriation of crip movement. Similar to how the movements of the bodies in the Americans with Disabilities Act protest may have been perceived as threatening and as spectacle, Cunningham also looks at this phenomenon of Presley himself. She also poses the idea that Presley's movement was always already endowed with crip movement through his uncontrolled and spasmodic hips, playing with ideas of brokenness within the physical lines of his body. In the installation, Cunningham provided documentary residue from her live performances, which included video, costumes and props. The artist had created jumpsuits of the style from Presley's 'Vegas Era' costumes, and Cunningham and her fellow dancers customised them with a crip aesthetic. These were set up on make-shift mannequins in the installation.

To emphasise this idea of disabling movement and the so-called disabled movement of Elvis Presley, Cunningham also set up a microphone and a small system karaoke with a playlist of Elvis songs that could be sung live by gallery visitors for the duration of the exhibition. By inviting visitors to engage directly with impersonation, it gave them the opportunity to literally step into their bodies and 'be with' disability (and Elvis) for a short time, while also having fun. Obviously, Elvis Presley has been cast into a radically new light through Cunningham's work, but she also has us question the so-called innocent nature of imitation. If we imitate Elvis, it's all in good fun, but if we imitate disabled bodies, this comes with a great deal more sensitivity and cautiousness. This work also suggests that Presley owes a great tribute to the pathologised disabled body to whom he too has unwittingly imitated and embraced, much like Tobin Siebers' concept of disability aesthetics itself – that disability has always been there, but it has never been marked as such. The movement of disability, then, is perhaps not as foreign or taboo as we may have previously thought.

Moving Towards New Views of Dwarfism

The art world benefits from hearing and experiencing the views of those who occupy the margins with their so-called outsider perspectives, and the artistic work by Corban Walker and curatorial interventions by myself contribute to destabilising the comfortable and so-called typical ways of moving through space and viewing art from only one height and positionality for non-disabled audiences. In this chapter, I have offered the reader insight into my journey as a person with dwarfism in a professional context, where the traditions of curating, particularly the convention of hang-height, have been particularly ableist and hard to combat. Contemporary dwarf artists Ricardo Gil, Laura Swanson and Corban Walker have been pivotal at centring the dwarf voice, vision and viewpoint in contemporary art practice and tradition. I owe my own curatorial experimentation and activism to their radical expertise. From curating artists Noëmi Laikmaer to Mowry Baden, Claire Cunningham and even Elis Presley into my projects, my approach has often mirrored that of Walker's artistic methodology, which oscillates between frustration and antagonism towards the audience, mixed with a desire to share in our difference with others. I encourage museums to show work by disabled and dwarf artists on a more regular basis, and I am encouraged by the progression of contemporary disability art in the past 10 years and the art world's reception of it, particularly in our pandemic era. While I think incorporating new protocols and consistent templates for hang-height in the museum is a long way off, I am hopeful that through our work, we will begin to shed light on our critical and spatial dwarf perspective, where new ways to orient to the world are not only enlightening but are transformative.

References

Biggers, A. (2019). What's the average height for women and how does that affect weight? *Healthline* [online]. https://www.healthline.com/health/womens-health/average-height-for-women. Accessed on June 29, 2023.

Dick, T. (2015). The flesh of the world review. *Border Crossings*, *34*(136), No. 4.

Hanson, S. P. (2011). A pavilion in the making: Behind Ireland representative Corban Walker's destabilizing Venice Biennale installation. *Modern Painter* [online]. http://205.234.169.45/news/story/37795/a-pavilion-in-the-making-behind%20.%C2%A0.%C2%A0.%20walkers-%20destabilizing-venice-biennale-installation/. Accessed on June 26, 2023.

Kruse, R. J. (2010). Placing little people: Dwarfism and the geographies of everyday life. In V. Chouinard, E. Hall, & R. Wilton (Eds.), *Towards enabling geographies: 'Disabled' bodies and minds in society and space* (pp. 183–198). Ashgate Publishing Ltd.

Mayo Clinic. (2023). *Dwarfism* [online]. https://www.mayoclinic.org/diseases-conditions/dwarfism/symptoms-causes/syc-20371969#:~:text=Dwarfism%20is%20short%20stature%20that,4%20feet%20(122%20cm). Accessed on June 29, 2023.

Walker, C. (2022, January 27). *Interview on zoom with Amanda Cachia.*

Chapter 2

Little Big Woman: Condescension – Sculpting the Oppositional Gaze

Debra Keenahan (Artist, Writer, Psychologist, Adjunct)

Big Anxiety Research Centre, UNSW, Australia

Introduction

> The big problem in art is being able to tell the story of your own village, while at the same time having your village become everyone's village. I want to be faceless. I hold a mirror to my face so that those who look at me see themselves and therefore I disappear. (Christian Boltanski, 1997)

The subject of my work is my lived experience. I endeavour for people who engage with the artworks to develop a sense of the world from my perspective – or as if they were me – a woman with achondroplasia dwarfism. The challenge is for my artworks to engage people such that they feel, experience and come to an understanding of the world as I do. I work with various mediums. Depending upon the aspect of my lived experience I want to communicate and the capacity of a medium to engage the predominant senses within that experience, these criteria will dictate the medium I choose for that work. I have another intention for my art practice and that is to challenge the artistic tropes of representation of the dwarf corporeality, which can be a further factor in both the choice of medium for a work and influence various artistic choices I make in the production of the work. A work that encapsulates this transactional dynamic in my art practice is the sculpture 'Little Big Woman: Condescension'. I will discuss the development and production of this sculptural work, thus exemplifying how I endeavour to 'tell the story of my own village' through my art practice. First, I will discuss the social framework of disability which encapsulates the development of disability identity – in particular, the dwarf identity. I will then describe and discuss the concept of *Relational Disability Aesthetics* as representing the *realpolitik* of disability – that is, the relational dynamics of disability. Works by the Spanish figurative sculptor Juan Muñoz will be described and critiqued as typifying the historical approach to the representation of the dwarf corporeality. The groundwork is then set for the account of my practice in the production of 'Little Big Woman: Condescension', showing how I endeavour for those who engage with this work to 'look at me' yet in doing so they 'see themselves'.

The Social-Relational Framework of Disability

The medical model has been predominant in the discourse of disability which emphasises the physical, intellectual and emotional differences between people as biologically determined and as such situated within the individual. Inherent to this medical perspective is the idea of comparison – as in being different from those who are considered to be the norm or average. However, critique of the simplicity of the medical model led to the development of more nuanced definitions that shifted focus to the contextual and relational dynamics which convey valuative judgements upon human biological characteristics. Thomas and Corker (2002, p. 18) describe this nuanced definitional shift as:

> ... (the) formulation that disability is the active and purposive social exclusion and disadvantaging of people with impairment, resides in its redefinition of disability as a social relational as opposed to biologically determined phenomenon. That is, disability becomes a product and oppressive quality of the social relationships that exist between people who are socially marked as having impairment and those who are marked as physically, sensorially and cognitively 'normal'.

This definition presents disability as a transactional phenomenon that does not negate or deny the existence or impact of differences upon people but rather shifts the focus to the act of negatively valuing those differences such that people with those differences are thought of and treated as lesser beings. In other words: 'The meaning of the body, thus the meaning of the self, emerges through social relations. We learn who we are by the responses we elicit from others' (Garland-Thomson, 2000, p. 334). For example, my dwarfism means I am visibly different from the majority of people, and I may take longer to perform some tasks. I may be required to exert more effort, employ an assistance tool or perform a task decidedly differently. However, it is in judgements which consider such differences as devalued and the negative treatment resulting from those judgements, that my social status has shifted to that of disabled. From my personal perspective, my dwarfism does not disable me. What disables me is peoples' attitudes to my dwarfism. Therefore, in my art practice, 'to tell the story of my own village', I represent and capture those nuanced actions and behaviours which communicate an attitude that my dwarf corporeality is judged negatively such that I am not treated as a moral equal.

The dynamic value-laden transaction between bodies, perceptions and emotions is debatably the essence of aesthetics. A predominant theme throughout the history of the visual arts is representation of the human body. As Noland (2014, p. 469) states: 'It could be claimed that all thinking about art begins with the Body' because not only is the body a central subject of art, but perceptions and feelings also have the capacity to be affected by art – which is essentially the relationship of embodiment to aesthetics. As such, the human body is instrumental in the perception and appreciation of art and particularly in the judgement of art representing the human body, with the representation of human bodies in art being reflective of judgements about those bodies. What is of particular interest to me is the role that the visual arts play in the politics of identity formation in which 'the body is a site where aesthetic and ethical considerations are deeply intertwined' (Irvin, 2014, p. 410). Through my work, when 'I hold a mirror to my face so that those who look at me see themselves', I endeavour to examine and reveal this interface and intertwining of aesthetics and ethical considerations. I do so by representing those situations, actions and conditions within social relations that I experience as having an oppressive quality and are thus disabling.

Relational Disability Aesthetics: Representing the **Realpolitik** *of Disability*

Historically, the discipline of aesthetics is characterised as a branch of philosophy focused upon the definition of art and beauty (Bennett, 2012). But aesthetics has been expanded and decolonised into a transdisciplinary inquiry utilising theories and critical practices aimed at usurping hegemonic oppressive power, tastes and ideas (Kelly, 2014). One such area of discipline expansion is Disability Aesthetics, a concept developed by Siebers (2005) to examine the role of disability in the visual arts. I have argued previously (2022, 2020, 2017), Disability Aesthetics, as currently configured, adheres to a restrictive definition of aesthetics as anchored in beauty and as such is focused on the literal physical representation of difference or materialist emphasis, rather than the socially dynamic transactions that disable people with impairment.

Initially, in examining the relationship between disability, art and aesthetics, Siebers (2002) critiqued how art changes viewers' perceptions of the art subject. He was intrigued with the paradox of an art object with apparent distortions and defects being judged as beautiful and admired, when a person manifesting the same characteristics could be judged as ugly and socially rejected – for example, the Greek sculpture *Venus de Milo* being representative of a woman with multiple amputations and facial disfigurement. Siebers (2010) describes Disability Aesthetics as:

> ...a critical concept that seeks to emphasise (sic) the presence of disability in the tradition of aesthetic representation... Disability aesthetics refuses to recognize the representation of the healthy body – and its definition of harmony, integrity, and beauty – as the

sole determination of the aesthetic. Rather, *disability aesthetics embraces beauty that seems by traditional standards to be broken, and yet is not less beautiful, but more so as a result.* (Siebers, 2010, p. 2)

The italicised statement illustrates Siebers' conceptually narrow and contradictory perspective on aesthetics. I make this critique on the basis that throughout his work, though Siebers makes no explicit statement, there is a sense he considers the visual arts as an avenue for improving the social standing of disabled people. I agree the visual arts can effectively challenge contemporary hegemonic perspectives on a swathe of social issues. However, by focusing upon aesthetics as an appreciation of the (disabled) body equating with 'beauty', Siebers is focusing on the physical condition of impairment. In doing so, disability is being presented within the framework of the medical model rather than the relational-social model of disability. Moreover, Siebers is adhering to the time-worn beautiful–ugly dialectic binary which potentially condemns Disability Aesthetics to, at worst, the status of an oxymoron and, at best, an expression of personal bias/preference and thus all too readily dismissed in a debate of subjective judgement traditionally privileging those without disability. Though there is ethical appeal in rejecting and thus nullifying the implication that subjects judged as ugly are thus undesirable, Moore (2014) effectively argues that rejection of the judgement of ugliness rarely correlates with a decrease in the very real negative consequences of being judged as such. Consequently, for Moore (2014), debate as to the location of subjects on the beautiful–ugly spectrum is ineffective in producing change in the treatment of those subjects. Rather, it is the examination of 'the experiential process involved in making judgements' about subjects that has the capacity of producing such social change. As such, in my artworks, I endeavour to capture this shift in representation of the corporeal difference of dwarfism to *focus on the act of judging* the corporeal difference of dwarfism. The 'act of judging' manifests in discriminating interactive dynamics that effectively casts the dwarf subject as the Other – succinctly described by Garland-Thomson (2002) as disabled people being 'visually conspicuous but politically and socially erased'.

The focus of Disability Aesthetics as currently conceptualised clearly needs to move away from the consideration of aesthetics as addressing the beautiful–ugly binary to the broader perspective of aesthetics as a transactive process. This shift, as suggested by Quayson (2014), would result in examination and representation of interactive dynamics which would also ensure Disability Aesthetics achieved its ethical intent of improving the social standing of the disabled. Moreover, extending Disability Aesthetics in this way means the representation of disability would broaden to encompass what Bourriaud (2002) describes as 'relational aesthetics' – an amalgam of aesthetics in which an artwork 'takes as its theoretical horizon the sphere of human interactions and its social context' (p. 160). From within a relational sphere, Disability Aesthetics would represent interactions, modes of social exchange and human relationships which capture and focus upon the dynamic 'act of judging' the subject as an Other. It is this relational dynamic that is instrumental in the formation of an identity of disability. Therefore, rather than considering disability as a matter of 'broken beauty', I describe such Relational Disability Aesthetics as:

> The experiential representation of an exceptional natural form that is surviving and thriving in a hostile environment. (2022, p. 40)

In effect, Relational Disability Aesthetics focuses upon the dynamics of subjectivity and intersubjectivity because, although the subject has 'an exceptional natural form', their disability is represented in the capture of the negative value judgement – 'a hostile environment' – communicated by the perceiver of the subject. Therefore, in developing and adhering to this concept of Relational Disability Aesthetics in my art practice, I invite viewers of my artworks to enter a self-reflective relationship with the work. In doing so, they experience ethical judgements about modes of embodiment manifest in social-relational dynamics that affectively define a person as an Other and thus disabled. Simply, viewers of my artworks 'behold the beholder' and in doing so experience the tension of being simultaneously the 'beholder' and the 'beheld' in an act of 'Othering' – or in Boltanski's words, 'look at me and see themselves'. Such a reflective and reflexive dynamic in artwork is what Hevey (1992) describes as the *Realpolitik* of Disability – 'the observed beginning their own observing'. This reflective and reflexive relational dynamic shift simultaneously changes the status of audiences from passive observers to interacting participants.

These dynamic relational shifts are best understood by illustrating a subtle challenge to the traditional practice of offering up a passive dwarf subject for visual consumption by the viewing audience as exemplified by works of the sculptor Juan Muñoz.

Viewing Dwarfism in 3D: Reflecting on the Consuming Gaze

The prolific Spanish sculptor Munoz produced 13 works that included figures of dwarfs. The earliest of these works, 'Dwarf with Three Columns' (1988) captures the relationship of the figure with the built environment – a consistent theme throughout Munoz's career (Martinou, 2012). Between 1995 and 1996, he produced seven works of a female dwarf, two of which repeat this subject-in-built environment theme (*Sara with* 'Billiard Table' – 1996; 'Sara with a Chair' – 1996). This theme of 'dwarf in an over-sized world' is an enduring visual trope focusing upon the different corporeality of the subject. However, his other works have an added dimension that reflect Munoz's attitude to his subject. Throughout his oeuvre, Munoz's figurative works emphasise dynamic capture of conversations and interactions – except for his subjects with dwarfism which he always represents as isolated figures. But the works of the female dwarf subject have a paradoxical prominence due to three elements. First, a mirror is contained in five works – an element not included in other Munoz sculptures – and the dwarf subject is 'interacting' with her reflection (e.g. 'Sara con Espejo' – 1996; 'Sara in Front of a Mirror' – 1996). These works Munoz describes as conceptual in intent:

> My characters sometimes behave as a mirror that cannot reflect...
> They are there to tell you something about your looking, but they
> cannot, because they don't let you see yourself. (Munoz in
> interview with Paul Schimmel, 2000; cited in Benezra & Viso,
> 2001, pp. 145–150)

The second prominent element is the 'personal' quality of naming the subject (Sara) – which does not occur with Munoz's other figurative sculptures. Third, in three of the works, Sara playfully lifts her skirt, displaying a coquettish quality. Such girlish titillation is unique among Munoz's work. So paradoxically, Munoz individualises and deeply personalises Sara in naming her while simultaneously presenting her as isolated and detached in her girlishness. Munoz is inviting the viewer's curious gaze but intentionally produces tension with a sense of self-reflective disquiet, as he states:

> There is something about their appearance that makes them
> different, and this difference in effect excludes the spectator from
> the room they are occupying...At one moment this is the means of
> reversal that has taken place. The spectator becomes very much
> like the object to be looked at, and perhaps the viewer is the one
> who is on view. (Munoz in interview with Paul Schimmel, 2000;
> cited in Benezra & Viso, 2001, pp. 145–150)

Consequently, Munoz is aiming to 'reverse the viewer's gaze' which effectively acknowledges the viewers as co-conspirators in their relationship to the artwork through their construction of the dwarf subject of the work (Keenahan, 2022). By Munoz wanting to reverse the viewer's gaze, though he may be endeavouring for the viewers to 'see themselves' as Boltanski says, the Otherness of the dwarf subject remains the focus of the work. So, though this reflective twist indicates a shift in Munoz's attitude towards his dwarf subjects, there remains a quality of 'enfreakment' (Hevey, 1992) in the sculptures. But the strategic manipulation of the viewer's gaze to focus upon their 'conspiratorial power' in the construction of the subject is a critical intersubjective dynamic that I argue is essential for the representation of Relational Disability Aesthetics. It is this critical intersubjective dynamic that is described by Boltanski in 'hold(ing) a mirror to my face so that those who look at me see themselves', which is the goal for my sculpture 'Little Big Woman: Condescension'.

Being Me and Sculpting the Oppositional Gaze

To represent the *Realpolitik* of the disability of dwarf identity formation – that is, 'being visually conspicuous but politically and socially erased' – my artistic challenge is to capture those nuanced interactions and microaggressions that communicate such erasure. Therefore, I immerse the viewer into my embodied experience, by reversing the focus upon and reflecting back the act of Othering.

So, though my work is about me and as such, 'I hold a mirror to my face', this strategic reflective shift means that figuratively and paradoxically, 'I disappear' because the focus of the work becomes the dynamic of me and people like me being 'politically and socially erased', but I am also positioning my work to be a site of resistance against such oppressive erasure. As such, my artworks represent 'aesthetic encounters' which are disabling. These encounters are interpretive acts which Saito (2014) describes as judgements that are aesthetically led and have considerable cumulative effects.

The haptic nature of sculpture makes the qualities of immediacy and materiality evident within tactile space (Mey, 2014). A figurative sculpture blurs the object–subject positioning because the sculpture achieves an object reality in becoming a 3D body itself (Mey, 2014). This shift in object–subject positioning, Mey claims, is the dynamic instrumental in viewers of a figurative sculpture experiencing the work as a 'dialogue of bodies' that raises 'questions regarding the locus of the aesthetic' (2014, p. 521). Paradoxically, it is the essential 'stillness' of sculptures that Getsy (2014) claims produces these provocations because the encounter is akin to a 'theatre of power relations' between active viewers and the passive sculpture. Consequently, because the sculptural medium is essentially corporeal and thus spatial and relational, Getsy (2014) describes the medium as more akin to an encounter with another person despite the scale of the work, but particularly if the work is one-to-one scale. Therefore, to effectively produce an aesthetic encounter experienced as disabling, I chose to make the work to scale. Furthermore, due to this performative quality of sculpture, I wanted the viewer of my work to be immersed into my perspective, so I aimed for the sculpture to engage with the viewer as if the viewer was me. Therefore, I chose to represent an interactional moment that communicates an attitude that the focus or target individual is not considered a moral equal but an Other – in what Melville (2014) describes as an asymmetry of power. The capture of such a social dynamic is consistent with Bourriaud's definition of relational aesthetics – 'in judging artworks on the basis of the inter-human relations which they represent, produce or prompt' (2002, p. 112, cited in Downey, 2007, p. 270).

The impact of a sculpture is its 'confrontational inertness' in a performative act (Getsy, 2014). Consequently, my artistic challenge was to produce a sculpture that represented a performative act that would engage the viewer so that the viewer became 'confronted' by the work. This sense of confrontation being in the performative act of the sculpture paradoxically visually consuming the viewer and thus the viewer being Othered.

Another dimension of sculpture is the capacity of viewers to circumambulate the work which Getsy (2014) claims puts the viewer in a position of superiority particularly regarding a figurative piece, through the freedom of their consuming gaze. Mindful of this dynamic, I intended that throughout the circumambulation of my work, viewers would have the sense of themselves as always being 'gazed upon' or 'stared at' – a constant in my lived experience of being visually conspicuous.

Staring is saturated with meaning because it is an emphatic response to another. But the meaning of the stare is context driven. The context in which the act of staring occurs can imbue the behaviour with various meanings from wonder, adoration and reverence to surprise, curiosity, hostility, domination – even disgust (Garland-Thomson, 2006). For my work, I wanted the viewers to experience themselves in accord with my lived experience, of being stared at negatively, that is, being 'looked down upon' (figuratively speaking). As such, the sculpture would manifest the dynamic of reverse audiencing by the dwarf subject of the sculpture through the manifestation of the oppositional gaze. Cachia (2014) describes the oppositional gaze as the traditionally objectified subject returning the gaze of the hegemonic viewer and thereby reclaiming agency.

I made 'Little Big Woman: Condescension' through the process of 3D printing [refer to Keenahan (2022) for a detailed account of the making of the sculpture] (see Figs. 2.1–2.3). The initial stage of the process required scanning of the subject to be printed – the subject being me. Figuratively, this was the stage at which I 'held a mirror to my face'. But, as I wanted to 'tell the story of my own village', I chose a stance very familiar to people with dwarfism – being spoken to 'as if' one is a child – that is, infantilisation. The subjective experience of infantilisation is of not being taken seriously and thus demeaned in social status (Pritchard, 2021). In other words, I wanted to capture the attitude of condescension, and in doing so, the viewers of the work 'look at me and see themselves' – or look at the figures and experience the sense of being 'spoken down to'.

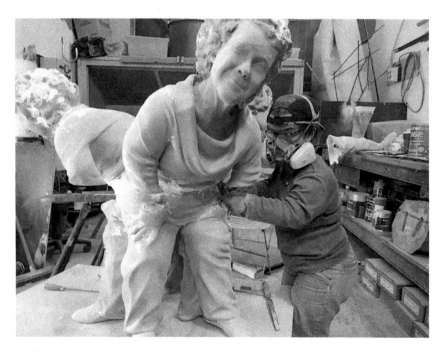

Fig. 2.1. Artist (Debra Keenahan) Working on the Sculpture. *Source:* Image - Robert Brindley ©.

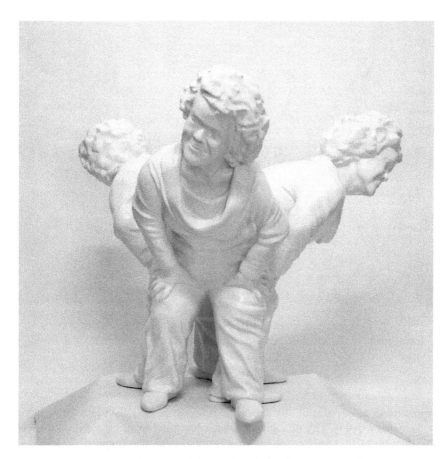

Fig. 2.2. 'Little Big Woman: Condescension'. *Source:* Artist - Debra Keenahan; Image - Robert Brindley ©.

To emphasise the intense intrusive power of the stare the work consists of a triple amalgam of the figure so that in circumambulating the work, the sculptured figures always 'look at' the viewers. To emulate classic Greco-Roman sculptures, I chose the work to be painted white. Finally, to literally have the work 'look down upon' viewers, the sculpture is mounted on a plinth 150 cm high so that the heads of the figures come 'face to face' with viewers of average height.

Conclusion: Telling the Story of My Village Is a Dialogue of Bodies

My purpose for 'Little Big Woman: Condescension' is for the work to represent my lived experience of being a woman with dwarfism. The focus of this

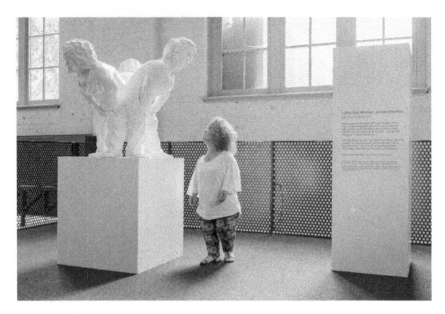

Fig. 2.3. Artist With 'Little Big Woman: Condescension' on Exhibition – Museum of Applied Arts and Sciences, Sydney, Australia.
Source: Image - Robert Brindley ©.

representation, but also all my artworks, is to act as a catalyst in a 'dialogue of bodies' (Mey, 2014). This dialogue about disabling experience is achieved through the disruption and subversion of conventional and stereotypical notions and perceptions pertaining to the representation of the corporeality of dwarfism. Instead, my strategy with Relational Disability Aesthetics is for those who interact with my work to experience 'the interpretive moment of social creation' of the conception of 'difference' (Shuttleworth & Meekosha, 2013). It is the social creation of 'difference' manifest in the act of erasure that is fundamental to the embodied experience and identity of disability.

Representing my embodied experience as a disabled person requires capturing the relational dynamics that communicate erasure or moral inequality in response to my dwarf corporeality. These dynamics coexist *with* the viewer of the work. Therefore, 'Little Big Woman: Condescension' aims to 'theatricalise' the space by blurring the object–subject positioning (Getsy, 2014). This theatrical blurring is achieved through reverse audiencing in which the sculptural subject 'stares at' the now-objectified viewer of the sculpture. Consequently, the locus of Relational Disability Aesthetics, as with the identity of disability, is dialogical, participatory and, as such, performative. In other words, with my art, I endeavour to 'tell the story of my village' by metaphorically making my work a 'mirror' reflecting the disabling dynamics I experience in response to my dwarfism.

References

Benezra, N., & Viso, O. (2001). Regarding beauty: A view of the late twentieth century. *The Journal of Aesthetics and Art Criticism, 59*(1), 145–150.

Bennett, J. (2012). *Practical aesthetics: Events, affect and art after 9/11*. IB Tauris.

Boltanski, C. (1997). *Phaidon*. https://www.artspace.com/magazine/art_101/book_report/christian-boltanski-phaidon-54886. Accessed on March 13, 2023.

Bourriaud, N. (2002). *Relational aesthetics [1998]*. Les presses du reel.

Cachia, A. (2014). Composing dwarfism: Reframing short stature in contemporary photography. *Review of Disability Studies: An International Journal, 10*(3, 4), 6–19.

Garland-Thomson, R. (2000). Staring back: Self-representations of disabled performance artists. *American Quarterly, 52*(2), 334–338.

Garland-Thomson, R. (2002). The politics of staring: Visual rhetorics of disability in popular photography. *Disability Studies: Enabling the Humanities*, 56–75.

Garland-Thomson, R. (2006). Ways of staring. *Journal of Visual Culture, 5*(2), 173–192.

Getsy, D. J. (2014). Acts of stillness: Statues, performativity, and passive resistance. *Criticism, 56*(1), 1–20.

Hevey, D. (1992). *The creatures time forgot: Photography and disability imagery*. Routledge.

Irvin, S. (2014). Body. In M. Kelly (Ed.), *Encyclopaedia of aesthetics* (pp. 410–414). Oxford University Press.

Keenahan, D. (2017). Friday essay: The female dwarf, disability, and beauty. *The Conversation*. https://theconversation.com/friday-essay-the-female-dwarf-disability-and-beauty-84844. Accessed on November 03, 2017.

Keenahan, D. (2020). Missing in action: Desire, dwarfism and getting it on/off/up—A critique and extension of disability aesthetics. In R. Shuttleworth & L. R. Mona (Eds.), *The Routledge handbook of disability and sexuality* (pp. 235–248). Routledge.

Keenahan, D. (2022). *Critical disability aesthetics-relational dynamics and the embodied experience of a female dwarf*. Doctoral dissertation, UNSW Sydney.

Kelly, M. (2014). Preface to the second edition. *Encyclopaedia of aesthetics* (pp. xxi–xxxvi). Oxford University Press.

Martinou, A. (2012). Juan Munoz sculptures. *Skarstedt Exhibitions Press Release*. https://www.skarstedt.com/gallery-exhibitions/juan-munoz/press-release. Accessed on March 05, 2023.

Melville, S. (2014). Gaze. In M. Kelly (Ed.), *Encyclopaedia of aesthetics* (pp. 150–152). Oxford University Press.

Mey, K. (2014). Sculpture: Overview. In M. Kelly (Ed.), *Encyclopaedia of aesthetics* (pp. 514–522). Oxford University Press.

Moore, R. (2014). Ugliness. In M. Kelly (Ed.), *Encyclopaedia of aesthetics*. Oxford University Press.

Noland, C. (2014). Embodiment. In M. Kelly (Ed.), *Encyclopaedia of aesthetics* (pp. 465–470). Oxford University Press.

Pritchard, E. (2021). *Dwarfism, spatiality and disabling experiences*. Routledge.

Quayson. (2014). Disability aesthetics. In M. Kelly (Ed.), *Encyclopaedia of aesthetics*. Oxford University Press.

Saito, Y. (2014). Everyday aesthetics. In M. Kelly (Ed.), *Encyclopaedia of aesthetics* (pp. 525–529). Oxford University Press.
Shuttleworth, R., & Meekosha, H. (2013). The sociological imaginary and disability enquiry in late modernity. *Critical Sociology*, *39*(3), 349–367.
Siebers, T. (2002). Broken beauty: Disability and art vandalism. *Michigan Quarterly Review*, *41*(2), 223–245.
Siebers, T. (2005). Disability aesthetics. *PMLA/Publications of the Modern Language Association of America*, *120*(2), 542–546.
Siebers, T. (2010). *Disability aesthetics*. University of Michigan Press.
Thomas, C., & Corker, M. (2002). A journey around the social model. In M. Corker & T. Shakspeare (Eds.), *Disability/postmodernity. Embodying disability theory* (p. 1831). Continuum.

Chapter 3

Where Are the Creative Opportunities for People With Dwarfism Lived Experience in Participatory Arts Funding?

Steph Robson (Creative Practitioner and Artist)

UK

Introduction

Where is *dwarf culture*? This was the question I asked on my blog, HelloLittleLady.com, in late 2010. Over 13 years later, as I started this chapter in late 2023, after another dwarfism awareness month, I am still scratching my head around this concept that keeps my mind occupied.[1] Thankfully, with my experience of accidentally falling into the world of art and culture with my own creative work and developing as a practitioner, I can finally articulate what I was trying to ask.

Arts and cultural activities, including people with dwarfism, appear to land in two distinct categories. The first focuses on raising awareness, educating and accessing wider social acceptance and inclusion. The second relates to where our bodies are objectified and ridiculed for mainstream consumption. Yet, from my observations of my creative art practice and activism with the dwarfism community over the past 4 years, there is an identity gap between the two. This identity gap allows dwarf people to engage and participate in arts and cultural activities on our terms. Furthermore, it allows them to engage in activities that seek to empower the dwarfism community to be creators and consumers of arts and cultural activities from our own lived experiences. We cannot do this alone, and this chapter argues that there is an urgent need for institutional support, time, funding, development, research and mentorship in creative opportunities for the dwarfism community. It proposes how this can be achieved, primarily through participatory arts, whether as professionals, individuals or groups.

---

[1]Dwarfism awareness month occurs every October.

Identifying the Identity Gap Between Educating and Objectification

We in the dwarfism community still rely on awareness raising and education to counter societal and cultural prejudice and ignorance. We are overjoyed to see role models included in mainstream programmes or dramas. Yet, my creative art practice and activism with the dwarfism community over the past five years have shown an identity gap between the two, an identity gap that provides opportunities for dwarf people to engage and participate in arts and cultural activities on our own terms, to engage in activities that empower the dwarfism community to be creators and consumers of arts and cultural activities of our own lived experiences, and importantly, explore what this 'identity' means to us individually and as a community.

How can this 'identity gap' of artistic expression and agency around the community's shared experiences be encouraged? The vehicle with which I propose this is through the medium of participatory arts. Yet, as the past five years have proved since my first self-funded exhibition, 'You're Just Little', there are challenges to this concept becoming a reality both within the community and externally.

I propose an urgent need for institutional support, time, funding, development, research and mentorship in creative opportunities for the wider dwarfism community. I also propose how this can be achieved, primarily through developing participatory art activities and the need for training and support as professionals, individuals or groups for members from the dwarfism community.

Has Awareness-Raising Had Its Time?

For years, many wonderful activists and role models have raised awareness of what it is like to live with dwarfism. Yet, time and time again, we see and hear of dwarf people being mocked or on the receiving end of negative attention that seems permissible to wider society. I have questioned why awareness-raising is not enough to counter this behaviour. Is there another way to do this that does not require us to call out disgraceful behaviour? How can we celebrate our lived experiences and direct the conversation of our lives on our terms and, in the process, heal (collective) trauma?

The problem with awareness-raising in 2023 begs the question, who is representation really for? From my observation of having blogged about my dwarfism journey for over 15 years, I have found representation appears to fall into two distinct categories. The first concerns educating average-height, non-disabled (and surprisingly other disabled) people about the challenges we face to access wider society acceptance and inclusion. Think of inspirational figures platformed on the front of magazines or newspaper articles. Or the latest disability campaigns, where they often talk about how they have 'overcome' some form of difficulty. I always remember the late, great Stella Young's TED Talk – 'I'm not your inspiration, thank you very much' (Young, 2014). A talk about how people perceived her as wonderful and offered her an award because she was disabled, or as Young's parents quipped, 'just for getting out of bed in the morning!' rather than for achieving anything in particular. As someone fortunate to be awarded a Young Woman of the Year award (many years ago), I became all too aware of how such accolades are rarely about the disabled person and the ensuing lack of attention or support once the shining lights of an award ceremony fade. We still find ourselves talking about the issues faced, the discrimination experienced and the prejudice and ignorance that continue.

I have struggled with this particular area of representation for some time. From the moment I started my blog, I was contacted by mainstream magazines, news and media outlets looking for stories of 'inspiration'. I refused to engage in this particular 'inspiration porn' type of work. It did not and still does not sit well with me. Why? Representations of our lives (or lack thereof) are filtered through (and continue to be so through) the lens of able-bodied, average-height gaze. What I could not articulate back in 2008/2009 at the start of my blogging journey, and well before that, was that this work and narrative is steeped in ableism. Awareness-raising and education have their rightful place. There are some fantastic role models (and I have a lot of respect for those) who do this work incredibly well in the community. Yet, personally and professionally, I am tired of educating society and still witnessing and facing the same structural challenges I mentioned above.

The second form of representation relates to where our bodies are objectified and ridiculed for mainstream consumption. The year 2010 was a different era; in the United Kingdom, we had a new Conservative-led coalition government that was hell-bent on reducing state support in the name of 'austerity'. The disabled community suddenly found themselves also having to contend with and defend themselves against the 'scrounger' narrative pushed by the British media with a much more callous benefit system. Not only did we have to contend with being 'inspirational', but we were also accused more or less of being a burden to society. You can imagine how conflicting this narrative was and continues to be manipulated for non-disabled political advantage and gain.

My awareness-raising experience included attempting to educate specific media staff at a well-known national radio station in London while on the BBC Extend scheme about why it was not a good idea for a comedy sketch to include the word 'midget'. This meeting, alongside attending a comedy night where the first comedian's sketch ruminated on how 'hilarious' it would be to 'put midgets in a ring and fight' to a raucously laughing Chiswick crowd who seemed to agree cemented my awareness and showed the blatant discrimination our bodies faced as a community. Furthermore, Warwick Davis's *Life's Too Short* (2011–2013) sitcom with Ricky Gervais, a comedian known for mocking disabled people, set a very uncomfortable line between laughing at oneself and what, as a viewer, felt like he was being laughed at.

Dwarfism was still very much the butt of mainstream comedian jokes, violence and contending with the simultaneous rise of being victims of mobile phone photography and being shared across social media 'for fun' (See Ellis, 2018; Pritchard, 2023). In 2019, British Comedian Jimmy Carr's 'Is a dwarf an abortion that made it' 'joke' which insinuated that our bodies are 'less than' or not fully human was aired with minimal backlash (Pritchard, 2019). YouTube had a 'Spot a Midget' channel, and Amazon's Midget Tossing t-shirts are further examples of the prejudice that our disability has experienced in mainstream society over the past decade and more. Our bodies are objectified. Our disability is ridiculed for mainstream consumption. People in our community can still be hired out for 'entertainment'. In every one of these actions and incidents, we are left voiceless.

Yet, from my observations, any dwarf voices platformed are still white, middle class who already had a substantial platform. However, this is not to dismiss their potential to raise awareness and foster a more positive representation of dwarfism. In 2022, influenced by Pritchard's (2021) research, Will Perry's Awareness Raising Campaign was launched on the BBC One show. Then there was Sinéad Burke's groundbreaking *Vogue* covers (2020, 2023) and Met Gala appearance (2019). It is difficult to assert whether these activities are genuinely groundbreaking or tokenistic exercises, as platforming and inclusion of dwarfism in arts and culture are still dependent on mainstream, non-disabled gatekeepers, including producers and magazine editors. Our faces are in the room more, yet we do not have a permanent seat, and inclusion still seems to rely on us trading on our (collective) trauma to be there in the first place.

Anecdotally, in 2023, I do believe there is more acceptance and intolerance to the objectification of dwarfism in society, at least in the media. The dwarfism community has experienced its first *Strictly Come Dancing* contestant with Ellie Simmonds MBE in 2022; she was also on the 2023 series of the British game show *The Wheel* and as a contestant for *The Great Comic Relief Bake Off* (2013). We have Kiruna Stamell in the daytime soap *Doctors* (2023–present), and Annabelle Davis has had a role in the soap opera *Hollyoaks* (2023). While it is fantastic to see strong characters on the screen and in print, and this type of representation is very much needed, I began to wonder if stories like mine and those of other dwarf people would ever be platformed.

Over the years, I have looked to the wider disability community for acceptance. Yet, from my observations, dwarfism is rarely seen or included in most discourse. I will never forget attending the online event on the *Ethics of Dwarfism and Humour* hosted by Disability Arts Cymru in July 2020 with Dr Erin Pritchard, Tamm Reynolds and Simon Minty, where the panel had to field questions such as the rightness of Channel 4's 'Undateables' from an audience made up of other disabilities. While the panel tried to raise awareness about dwarfism, it felt like a massive missed opportunity for the wider disability community to learn, support and help further the much-needed conversation.

These experiences all started to build a picture for me of the lack of dwarf stories in the arts and culture of our lived experiences. Generally, we do not appear to have a say in discourse unless we are an inspiration, scrounger, awareness-raising figure, the 'token' under-represented group in the room or objectified for someone else's political gain. So, has awareness-raising had its day? The question that needs to be posed – or at least thought about – is whether awareness-raising has been at the expense of creating opportunities that allow the dwarfism community to gain self-actualisation, agency and a sense of self. Or, how can we create art or cultural opportunities that allow us to make sense of our lived experiences on our own terms rather than to justify our place in society? That is not for the consumption and education of the non-disabled and where we do not have to trade on our collective community (and personal) trauma to gain access to a space at the table.

Awareness-raising is constrictive. It relies on the person with dwarfism to relay their trauma to gain access to support or inclusion and identity. We need space to develop our narratives and agency in arts and culture that does not rely on shoehorning ourselves into how society prefers to digest our shared identity. Yet this is the prevailing narrative and expectation people with dwarfism (and disability) face.

The Struggle to Articulate and Accept One's Identity and Agency

It has been a lifetime's work to accept my identity as a dwarf person. It has not been easy. It has been an uphill battle to articulate my lived experiences in a society that actively dismisses, asks me to reject and belittles their enormity. I was constantly told, 'You're normal', 'you're just little' or told I was 'too sensitive' when trying to talk about how I was laughed at walking down the street or facing discrimination or assault. It left me voiceless and confused about where to find my space in the world. Yet, I have always been motivated by creating community and connection. In my early university days, I established the first online support group for people with Russell Silver Syndrome in 1999.[2] Members from all over the world joined, and for the first time, others and I had control over what was discussed without the prying ears and eyes of parents and medical professionals. The journey to permit myself to express myself would take another decade.

This came about when I took a short non-fiction writing course in 2008. One of the tasks was to set up a blog and write our first post. I wrote what I knew about. My own lived experience of being laughed at while walking down the street. Hearing 'Hello, Little Lady!' shouted at me across a busy Asda [British supermarket chain] car park by an excited toddler seeing a small woman (and being pulled away by his very embarrassed mum) sealed the fate. I set up my blog with that moniker not long thereafter.

I blogged anonymously to start with. I had been involved with the wider dwarfism community in the mid-2000s for a few years and had become very aware of the political climate I found myself in and was wary of putting my head above the parapet. I had also been through traumatic experiences that I needed the space to process for myself without having to deal with the reactions of people who knew me.

Due to the anonymity, I was often contacted and asked if I was either the late Bev or Jazz Burkitt from the *Small Teen, Bigger World* (2011) documentary. Bev Burkitt was hugely influential in my activism. I will always remember a spirited conversation at my first Restricted Growth Association sessions in 2006. That conversation, around how the abuse we faced would not be tolerated for other minority groups, started me on the path to being able to articulate the prejudice,

---

[2]A form of dwarfism.

ignorance and discrimination I face, and that it was ok to do that. These two amazing ladies were instrumental in changing the conversation around dwarfism and how we are treated by society in the 2000s.

I loved those early blogging days. The internet was a much friendlier place for people to flourish freely. Personally, that freedom to write gave me a much-needed outlet. Professionally, I found myself promoting opportunities for various media outlets and noting when dwarfism appeared in the media and arts. It was in 2010 that I first asked the question, 'Where is dwarf culture?' It would take another decade before I was able to answer this question.

Becoming a Participatory Artist and Creative Activist

In 2016, I came out of the blogging closet. I remember one person saying, 'It's you?!' with utter surprise. I was under the impression people thought the author behind the posts had achondroplasia.[3] Yet, what HelloLittleLady.com showed was that while medical issues may differ between different forms of dwarfism, we all share very similar experiences with how society reacts to our bodies.

My journey into participatory practice came about by chance. I was invited to join the ArtWorks-U participatory network meeting at The National Glass Centre in Sunderland by my former MA Radio course leader, Professor Caroline Mitchell, at the University of Sunderland in 2017. These meetings, attended by participatory artists across Sunderland, began a journey into a world I had no idea existed. Again, people would cross my path to help me place where I am today with my practice. I would like to mention the artist Kathryn Barnett. We bonded over our shared frustration with disability exclusion in the creative field, and they were instrumental in starting me on the path to being able to call myself an artist.

After one meeting, I mentioned an idea I had for an exhibition. She asked for a proposal, and a few months later, 'You're Just Little' was exhibited at the Spectrum Cultural Hub in County Durham in 2018.[4] I did not realise the enormity that the exhibition would have, professionally and personally. 'I just want to put some photos from my height, at my height, on a gallery wall' was how I put it. In reality, it was another instance of me taking space where, traditionally, dwarfism is objectified. Kathryn suggested the participatory element (which would inform my practice moving forward). I invited the dwarfism community to share a wall with my exhibition by sending photos from their perspective, too. I was surprised by the response to the call out. Over 50 photos were sent in from members of the dwarfism community in the United Kingdom, United States, New Zealand and Australia. When hanging these photos on the wall, I realised that I had never seen another dwarf person's perspective from my perspective/similar height in an art setting before. Most of the reaction from (average-height) people who attended was 'I didn't realise', to which I would reply, 'I can write a thousand words about the difficulties I face, but a photo shows this clearly'.

---

[3]Achondroplasia is the most common form of dwarfism.
[4]The Spectrum Cultural Hub was an Arts learning project based in Dawdon, Co. Durham, with studios, project & gallery spaces.

My journey to becoming an artist and creative activist began. I did not have the vocabulary or even the awareness to articulate this. To me, artists were fine art painters or weird and wonderful contemporary art exhibitions seen at The Baltic Centre for Contemporary Art in Gateshead. Activists were people who broke windows. Yet, new opportunities resulting from this exhibition would challenge my perceptions of both. In 2019, I found my people as part of the first cohort of the UNION Arts – a sector-based, year-long course for emerging community artists and activists. That first weekend at ChapelFM in Leeds gave me the language, the context and the confidence to start claiming this identity as a creative activist.[5] Crucially, it took me out of the North East of England to meet people who were also doing amazing work for their communities.

Being awarded a Creative Development Fellowship by Sunderland Culture the same year to explore running participatory podcasting for the dwarfism community was exciting and terrifying. I was unaware of any other event like that outside of the convention sphere. I knew getting the community to trust that the workshops would be safe for participants to attend would be an uphill battle. The first workshop was 'What's Your Story' held in Leeds in October 2019. Despite lots of promotion and reaching out to people, only one local participant turned up.

I began to wonder if I was ahead of my time. In reality, the lack of trust in an environment that traditionally mocks dwarf people and the prominence of issues regarding accessibility and financial costs to the participant provided a sharp lesson as a practitioner to the effort and challenges it takes to encourage participation. The second workshop, which was supposed to be held in Sunderland, was cancelled due to a lack of interest from the community. The interest was mainly from healthcare professionals wanting to attend for their specific agendas. One academic said they 'were working their way up to the top, to talk to Tom Shakespeare', which was not exactly the confidence-inducing validation I was looking for at the time.[6]

Turning the Corner With Participatory Engagement With the Dwarfism Community

Ironically, the pandemic in 2020, horrific as it was for the dwarfism and wider disability community, provided opportunities for those of us who had adopted technology for working and expression long before the mass workforce. Suddenly, the disability community found ourselves at the centre of being asked how to use technology for engagement and how we could use this to help organisations reach the masses. Funding, fuelled usually by the prevalent placed-based funding model of more recent years, was made available to work with communities online for artists. UNION Arts was one of those funders who asked our cohort (and to

---

[5]Chapel FM is a community radio station based in Leeds, England.
[6]Professor of Disability research.

provide us a chance at what it was like to apply for a commission) to explore new ways of working with communities through the pandemic.

WayFinders was one of the commissions funded, a participatory podcast project that engaged with women from the dwarfism community over six workshops to talk about the more humourous aspects of their lived experiences of our disability. This time, I reached out to potential participants personally and fielded any questions or reservations they had, and that there was no pressure on them to speak. The delivery was better suited online as it allowed people with dwarfism to gather together without having to travel. Participants joined from Orkney to Southampton and in between.

While I had designed the workshops around the themes of humour and comedy, there was a much richer conversation around the daily prejudice and ignorance that our community faces and the sharing of wisdom and humour in the encounters we find ourselves brought into. It was here that the participants, by joining the workshops, showed the community that it is possible to control how our stories are told through co-creation and permitting ourselves the space to talk. From this experience, I could articulate ideas into what I now know to be projects and practice. Sadly, the funding and promises of more hybrid engagement disappeared once the world opened again. I also experienced pushback from within the dwarfism community itself.

Discrimination and Acceptance From Within the Dwarfism Community

The path to creating participatory engagement for the dwarfism community has not been easy. Yes, there is a case to be made to funders and organisations. Still, the most challenging aspect of this journey has been the reactions, attitudes and indifference I have experienced directly from within the community. There has always been an element of 'you're not a proper dwarf' being said to people like myself with proportionate forms of dwarfism from the achondroplasia community. This internal discrimination means those of us with proportionate dwarfism feel stuck in the middle – of not being 'dwarf enough' but still being on the receiving end of ignorance and prejudice because of our medical conditions.

It is a strange, anchorless place to reside. I wonder, at times, why I feel I have received very little acknowledgement for my contribution to raising awareness around dwarfism. Hearing a prominent community member state that they prefer to 'do things behind the scenes rather than be an activist', despite attending the funded workshops brought about because of my activism, was disheartening. Granted, this response could be due to their internalised fear of drawing more attention to themselves than they already receive as a dwarf person. Their reaction shows the nuanced and political path we have to navigate to gain wider societal acceptance and adhere to the inspiring, awareness-raiser role many of us are foisted with. Witnessing parts of the community being very happy to use my skills to either platform themselves or copy some of my concepts without attribution has been one of the more distressing aspects of trying to find my sense of place and identity within the community.

This sense of isolation, I feel, is because there is a lot of work to be still done for proportionate dwarfism to gain acceptance (and acknowledgement) in the wider dwarfism community (and be recognised as someone with dwarfism by wider society). Mainly, I attribute the response, or lack thereof, to the inherent distrust of engaging in arts and cultural activities due to how the community has historically been objectified. Our community has not had the cultural investment to own our collective identity beyond the above-mentioned objectification, education and awareness roles.

Navigating Local and National Communities, Politics and Gatekeepers in the Arts in the United Kingdom

My apparent success in receiving funded opportunities also left me open to resentment from other local participatory artists when awarded funding for these workshops. The competitiveness of funding and a perception of lack of arts training, or more so a Fine Arts degree, has left me questioning my ability to take space in the participatory field, the wider art world or whether to call myself an artist at all. This, combined with the competitive landscape within which current participatory funding models operate, puts you at the behest of institutional and organisational gatekeepers. Those who decide which under-represented groups will be platformed for the mainstream spotlight are the tip of the iceberg of the challenges faced by a creative practitioner. My piece, as part of the 2021 'Disability and the Politics of Visibility' series at Durham Book Festival of 'tired of trading on my trauma to gain access to space and place', saw my frustrations with the sector start to emerge.

Practising as a Practitioner

I have been very fortunate to have had access to support, mentorship and funding, for which I am incredibly grateful. There have been people in the arts and cultural sector who have been nothing but encouraging in developing me as a practitioner – such as Kathryn Barnett and Professor Caroline Mitchell (ArtWorks-U), Laura Brewis (Sunderland Culture/We Make Culture), Adrian Sinclair and Sara Domville (UNION Arts) and New Writing North, Lizzie Coombes and Jo Verrent as part of my Arts Council England Develop Your Creative award. Dr Erin Pritchard has also been instrumental in validating and championing my work. Author and multi-discipilnary artist Lisette Auton, and disabled artist, Llady Kitt who both personify inclusion, platforming and who are incredible role models for fellow disabled artists. I would also like to include Vici Wreford-Sinnot here. A passionate disabled writer, director and campaigner for cultural equality, Vici has consistently included and supported my place in the art space and they are an inspiring role-model for my own practice and feeling seen these past 4 years.

Yet, there have been many challenges and frustrations with practising as a participatory practitioner. Working with communities that have experienced trauma invariably triggers your own trauma, and it has been a lesson in itself on how to implement or know how to put support in place for all involved.

The balance of finding external participatory projects and commissions with the wish to develop your own community projects reflects the wider artistic ecology within the United Kingdom, where artists engage with projects to help fund their wider practice. Yet, as a disabled practitioner, it became acutely obvious that I would have to choose between commissions and/or a part-time job (to bring in income) at the expense of pursuing my practice due to varying energy levels, access issues and relying on word of mouth to prove my capability as a practitioner.

This field is neither financially stable nor a viable source of income. You are constantly on the treadmill of looking for projects and applying for funding (a thankless, unpaid task as a freelancer). The stress of all the above over the past few years, especially with personal health issues and family challenges, led to hospitalisation with pneumonia in 2023. Facing my mortality while in hospital and the subsequent reflection on the circumstances that brought me to being hospitalised left me feeling angry and conflicted in pursuing this type of cultural work, or at the very least, how I can do this without experiencing complete burnout. The harsh realities of the arts and cultural environment I find myself in (as do other creative practitioners) in the United Kingdom in 2023, with the predominance of participatory placed-based practice, left me wondering if it is worth risking my physical and mental health any further.

What Is Dwarf Culture?

We need the space, time and resources to answer this question fully. We must be given the tools to create a pipeline of dwarf talent to engage in artistic practice, tools and skills that build engagement (and the confidence) to access mainstream arts and culture opportunities as creative professionals. This can include more mainstream roles in TV, publishing, or more engagement with the arts, where we can be platformed and published readily. Put simply, we need the space, time and tools to figure out what this looks like and how we wish to shape this engagement for the future.

Despite my evolution as a creative practitioner and emerging body of participatory work, as we now enter into 2024, I would argue that as a community, we have yet to acquire the language to be able to articulate or feel like we have permission to take ownership of how we want to engage with the world informed by our disability, creatively. The predominance of placed-based funding in participatory arts has not helped the cause. Granted, I still have a lot to learn about funding, but it is frustrating when it feels like most doors are shut tight because predominant funding requirements do not accommodate art creation outside this placed-based model.

Making the Case for Dwarf Culture

It is still possible to make a case for dwarf culture in 2024, but first, we must question who it is for and its intended outcome for the dwarfism community.

The answer to these questions, I suspect, will evolve over time and with investment. We need to ensure that all sections of the community are included. That we are given the tools to navigate historical politics (and representations) and a willingness for all to sit at the table to start the conversation about our shared identity anew. From my practitioner experience, there has been an inherent tension in how to marry participatory practice and my own to articulate this.

What I realise now, from having recently completed my Develop Your Creative Practice, 2024 (a grant awarded by Arts Council England), where I created a set of dwarf concept photos to explore the narratives and themes around the lived experience of dwarfism called *Taking Space* (Robson, 2024), is that my work has been an attempt to model and create opportunities for dwarf culture to exist. What struck me when photographing the hugely talented performance artist Alice Lambert was how much I focused on placing her front and centre. It was amazing to have the opportunity to create a body of work from a dwarfism perspective, and it has gone some way in restoring my faith in the profession. To boldly 'Take Space' as a dwarf person in a sector or society where our lived experiences are front and centre, to create our own culture unapologetically. To inhabit that 'identity gap' I identified earlier in this chapter.

Today, support and representation for the dwarfism community are restricted to several charities that either focus on sport or are rooted in awareness-raising and education, and they do this very well. However, in 2024, no arts organisations are available specifically for the dwarfism community. For dwarf culture to emerge, this needs to be remedied. It is not enough to be included within the wider Disability Arts community, nor would I argue for its inclusion to be bolted onto the existing support organisations in the dwarfism community. Research undertaken as part of the You're Just Little exhibition (Robson, 2018a) supports this call to action. The data revealed that 86% of participants felt unrepresented in the arts. Ninety-three per cent said better representation of dwarfism was needed in the arts. Comments from participants show the clear need for the inclusion of dwarf people in artistic practice.

> We're still the object in art. We're never the creator. Where are the exhibits BY little people?
>
> I simply have never seen an art exhibit tailored for people with dwarfism.
>
> People with dwarfism to be encouraged to participate in art. Art projects to include those with dwarfism.
>
> We need to be shown as just as capable of creating quality art as we are of being quality art (Robson, 2018b).

We have a specific set of lived experiences needing recognition, acknowledgement and investment. Firstly, to help the dwarfism community develop trust in engaging in artistic practice and arts and cultural activities. My work shows an inherent mistrust by dwarf people walking into art settings like galleries and museums for fear of how we will be treated once in the building, let alone deal with how we may be represented on a gallery wall or engaging in practice.

It is about developing skills and confidence to engage in participatory arts without apologising or dismissing our trauma and identities to be able to do so. To have fun and connect and not to have the burden and responsibility of educating the masses. I believe we must use participatory arts to create and support future artists in developing dwarf culture.

Conclusion

This chapter asks where the creative opportunities for people with dwarfism lived experience in participatory arts funding are. From my work and engaging with the community, I realised that I want to see the art of my own lived experience (and others with dwarfism) reflected back to us, but we need investment. In people, in skills, in understanding the community's long, traumatic past and the wariness of accessing and engaging in arts and cultural spaces for our community. That we are allowed to 'take space' creatively, we need the sector to move away from the reliance on placed-based funding to focus on the artists who desperately want to create and make change for their communities that is long term and sustainable.

Organisations and funders need to earn our trust – and fund and pay artists fairly for the contribution we give to the sector. The dwarfism community needs a broader cultural representation away from 'achondroplasia-centric' representation to include all forms of dwarfism, whether disproportionate or proportionate. We need to hear more women's voices, the global majority and the identities of our rich community. Our community needs creative nurturing of dwarf culture – to develop identity, voice and agency within arts and cultural spaces. We must be ambitious in the scale of thought, change and work we create. Who's with me?

References

Disability and the politics of visibility. *Durham Book Festival 2021* [online]. https://www.youtube.com/watch?v=Kjeu5Ec6M28&t=17s. Accessed on December 14, 2023.
Ellis, L. (2018). Through a filtered lens: Unauthorized picture taking of people with dwarfism in public spaces. *Disability & Society*, *33*(2), 218–237.
Life's Too Short. (2011–2014). British Broadcasting Corporation.
Pritchard, E. (2019). Jimmy Carr's dwarfism 'joke' is a reminder people like me are still treated as just a punchline. *Huffington Post* [online]. https://www.huffingtonpost.co.uk/entry/jimmy-carr-dwarfism-joke_uk_5d0cbdece4b0aa375f4b1362. Accessed on April 04, 2024.
Pritchard, E. (2021). *Dwarfism, spatiality and disabling experiences*. Routledge.
Pritchard, E. (2023). *Midgetism: Exploitation and discrimination of people with dwarfism*. Routledge.
Robson, S. (2018a). You're just little exhibition web page [online]. https://www.hellolittlelady.com/youre-just-little/. Accessed on December 14, 2023.

Robson, S. (2018b). You're just little exhibition research web page [online]. https://www.hellolittlelady.com/youre-just-little/exhibition-research/. Accessed on December 14, 2023.

Robson, S. (2024). Taking space – Develop your creative practice, funded by arts council England. https://www.hellolittlelady.com/develop-your-creative-practice-taking-space/. Accessed on January 27, 2024.

Young, S. (2014). I'm not your inspiration, thank you very much [online]. https://www.ted.com/talks/stella_young_i_m_not_your_inspiration_thank_you_very_much. Accessed on December 14, 2023.

Chapter 4

It's Behind You: How Equity and an Education Made Me More Than Just a Suit Filler

Alice Lambert (Performance Artist and Actor)
UK

Erin Pritchard (Senior Lecturer in Disability Studies)
Liverpool Hope University, UK

Introduction

The performing arts have not always been kind to people with dwarfism, and the idea of making a career from it can be seen as an impossible task. However, Alice Lambert has managed to carve a career as a Performance Artist and Actor, as well as a teacher of Drama. In this chapter, Alice explores her own experiences, including the tough times and painful moments. She openly explains that early in her career, she was naive and completely blindsided by the initial buzz of performance. As a result, she did not question her rights or if she was being respected as an equal. While she will openly tell anyone who asks, 'Yes, I have done Snow White and the Seven Dwarfs', in the first part of this chapter, she unpicks her experience and explains for people to understand why she would never do that role ever again. Alice then argues that if we want to see changes for people with dwarfism in the industry, we need to look at the whole spectrum of performance and dwarfism. In the second part, Alice shows that through time, hard work and perseverance, how she has created the career she has now. Alice explains how the narrative which runs through her work has always got some acknowledgement of dwarfism and equal rights. Occasionally, she will approach this with a big political gesture, telling a story through her work and acknowledging who we are and what needs to change. Other times, it may just be a subtle motif that flows through some contemporary dance.

In the Beginning

While Alice's educational background is impressive and has certainly aided in her building a respectable career in the performing arts, it has not been an easy journey. Alice describes her educational background as horrific due to a mixture of bullying and long absences due to extended periods spent in hospital. Growing up, Alice underwent numerous operations to try and correct her bowed legs, a common feature of achondroplasia. She also experienced a lot of bullying from other pupils, especially when in high school. It is common for pupils with dwarfism to experience bullying (Ktenidis, 2022). Experiencing bullying is socially and culturally produced and therefore not a product of achondroplasia, but rather of society. Despite wanting an education, as a result of the bullying, Alice left school with no qualifications.

In 2012, Alice started to attend a UK-based association for people with dwarfism with her average-sized husband and two children. The association was founded in 2012 as a support organisation for people with dwarfism in the United Kingdom. Until recently, the patron of the association was a dwarf actor, who co-owns a casting agency for tall and short people. Alice explains how she found out she had been put on the agency's books without her knowledge when she got an audition for the 2018 sequel *Mary Poppins Returns*. 'I had been going to [name of association]. In the early days, it seemed like a nice group of people. [Patron and co-owner of the agency] had put me on their books without me knowing. They called me up to talk about this role for Mary Poppins Returns, and I said, 'but I'm not even on an agency yet', and they were like, 'Oh, well, we'll pick you up as part of [name of agency]'. It is something within the arts. I did not think about that, I just thought 'You've just taken my information and set me up for an audition without really clarifying with me''.

Alice's role involved being a double for one of the child actors, which also involved some stunts. She states that the agency never told the film crew about Alice's limitations, which meant that she was expected to do certain physical activities. I soon noticed that there were cracks with the agency. They never really told the film crew of my physical limitations. So, they were expecting me to be able to just jump off of things and do certain physical activities that I just thought, *no, I can't actually do that*. The other people I was working with had a completely different type of dwarfism to me for a start. They were all in proportion. They did not have any spinal, shoulder or leg issues, so they could do what they wanted to do physically. Whereas I was a bit more limited, and I really had to kind of stand my ground a few times and just say, 'There are certain things you want me to do, I'm not going to be able to do it, it is actually, physically impossible to do'. While dwarfism is mostly associated with short stature, other secondary conditions associated with achondroplasia include spinal stenosis, which can cause mobility impairments. As a result, people with achondroplasia are told to avoid certain physical activities, such as jumping.

After she finished working for Mary Poppins Returns, Alice left the agency and joined another, which claims to 'be home of 400+ extreme height actors'. According to Alice, this agency is substantially better at managing and looking after its members. Despite leaving the previous agency, Alice recalls still being offered roles through them. 'Even after telling [previous agency] that I did not want to be with them anymore, they still kept contacting me. They were still contacting me with certain jobs they wanted to send me on, which I just kept saying, 'I've told you to please take me off of your books". While both casting agencies are providing a service for the entertainment industry and providing short and tall actors with employment, their premise is similar to the freak show. While not all of the casting will be for derogatory roles, the focal point is still the actor's stature, which is used for the audience's amusement.

While at the second agency, Alice did a round of pantomime, which she believes she was compelled into doing as it is often romanticised by other dwarf actors, who Alice recalls saying, 'Oh, honestly, Alice, it's brilliant, you know it. It gives the power back to you, and it's all about empowering you. And it's about us taking this role that was meant for us'.[1] However, it is hard to conceive how the power has been given back to them when the representation of the seven dwarfs is controlled by average-sized writers. How the seven dwarfs are presented within the pantomime has been argued to be based upon disabling humour, which encourages the audience to laugh at their stature (Pritchard, 2022). The only reason that a person with dwarfism fulfils the role is because of their stature, which Alice refers to as 'suit fillers'. A suit filler is an actor with dwarfism whose sole purpose is to use their stature for entertainment purposes. It is their physique that is of importance as opposed to their acting ability. Thus, it is important to consider how the characters are depicted based on their stature.

According to Alice, in the pantomime, a dwarf actor is a suit filler who does not get that many lines, which further suggests that their stature is the main focus. 'Maybe you will get two or three in the whole of the show if you are lucky and you get paid half the wage of the other characters, because you are just these token seven performers that everyone just wants to see. Children are excited to see you, and everyone is hyped up to see you, but ultimately you do not have to do much to make them laugh, which is even worse, because basically, they are already laughing at you as soon as you come on stage, because you are just standing there being yourself [a person with dwarfism], and that is funny to them. You have not even cracked a joke or done something comical in your movement. The audience is just laughing at your body. What then, is the difference between this and the original P.T. Barnum? When people find out, "Oh, there are going to be actually seven small people playing these roles" rather than children, or whatever, then it is like, "Oh, brilliant! Let's get tickets for that because we were actually allowed to then see seven of them [dwarfs] in one." Go and laugh and joke, and it is all okay, "cause it is Panto", and the audience has been given that licence and freedom to do that'.[2]

---

[1] A pantomime is a stage-based form of entertainment, often shown over the Christmas season. According to Sladen (2017), it is a staple of British Christmas tradition and an important part of the United Kingdom's cultural and theatrical landscape.
[2] 'Panto' is short for 'pantomime'.

It is important to recognise that the pantomime version of *Snow White and the Seven Dwarfs* is not based on the original Grimm fairy tale, but rather Disney's 1937 version of the story (Pritchard, 2022). Watson (2020) argues that Disney's version of the story follows the conventions of the freak show, which constructed dwarfs as oddities and acceptable to laugh at. Alice compares being in the pantomime with the Victorian freak show. Probably, the most well-known freak show owner is P.T. Barnum (1810–1891). Barnum's most famous freak show performer was Charles Stratton (1838–1883), aka General Tom Thumb. The purpose of the freak show was to display those with extreme bodily differences, such as people with dwarfism or gigantism, for audiences to stare in wonder at. The freak show is described as 'the formally organised exhibition of people with alleged and real physical, mental, or behavioural anomalies for amusement and profit' (Bogdan, 1988, p. 10). Thus, when the dwarfs have minimal dialogue but audiences still find their presence amusing, it is their dwarfism they are being entertained by and are often laughing at.

As Alice has a genuine passion for performing, initially, she recalls 'feeling the buzz of live theatre'. While Alice enjoys performing in front of a live audience, she began to realise that they were laughing at her dwarfism when she started interacting with audience members after the show. 'It was not until sort of part way through that I started to think, especially, when people who were in the audience say, 'Oh, we loved you out there. You were so funny'. I think I did not actually do that much, that was funny. I sneezed a few times, and that was it. They would come to the stage door after the show, but I realised that they just wanted to meet 'a dwarf'. The realisation that you are not being represented as a performer but rather your dwarfism is being paraded for the amusement of others can impact your emotional well-being.

I hit a really low point in where I was. I was so far from home. I wanted to quit, but at the same time, I thought, *Oh, what do I do?* I had just committed myself to this six-week run and was concerned about what would happen if I suddenly quit. I wish now that I had just done it because, looking back now, the worst that would happen is, they say right, you will never do another panto with us again. I realise now that it did not matter if they said that, as I never want to do another pantomime. When it comes to any of my future work if that was to have ever come up and say, 'Oh, is it true you walked out on this? Why?' I realise now I could have easily explained why I did. There were many times I would ring my husband crying and he just said, 'Just come home' or 'I'll come there and I'll help you back', and 'You know you don't have to do it'. I think complete naivety on my part was what was making me stay thinking, 'Oh, but I don't want to look bad'.

Unfortunately, despite the emotional toll, Alice felt that she could not speak out about how people with dwarfism were being treated within the pantomime. From Alice's experiences, including being backstage, she claims that there is a lot of bullying that goes on towards people who want to speak up. I just find it absolutely devastating. They are trying to silence those who want change. She recalls how backstage, such as in the dressing rooms, you could not talk about anyone, such as activists, who have a negative opinion about *Snow White and the*

Seven Dwarfs. You are not allowed to talk about anyone that is an advocate for dwarfism and trying to push for more positive roles. While the dwarf performers can convince themselves that they are providing audiences with enjoyment, it is the basis for that enjoyment that they can try to ignore.

Unfortunately, when dwarf actors try to silence others from speaking out, they are not only hampering equality for themselves but for anyone with dwarfism. We had a lady called [name] because we were in [place], where she lived. I had heard this story, but obviously, it was told to me in a negative way. It was announced that the local theatre's annual pantomime would be Snow White and the Seven Dwarfs, and she was trying to fight to get it cancelled and give her reasons why. We got told something from a producer that she was planning on sabotaging a performance, and this was before we had even done our first performance yet. Two cast members with dwarfism were interviewed with her, and they were trying to justify their reasoning behind why they do it. I believe she has two children, who also have dwarfism, which means she is fighting for advocacy for them as well. The two dwarf entertainers said, 'Oh, well, you know, this is something our children could do, and this is something that's good for them to see that we can do these things'. They were completely oblivious to the social repercussions the representation has, as well as the fact that people with dwarfism are capable of other things.

It is not only the performance that hinders equality for people with dwarfism but the continual backlash against activists often by dwarf entertainers. Unfortunately, the media often give dwarf entertainers a platform to speak out in a way that suggests they are speaking on behalf of all people with dwarfism (Pritchard, 2023). The only interaction the majority of general society has with dwarfism is through the media. As the media already perpetuates problematic stereotypes of dwarfism, having dwarf entertainers defend these representations suggests to general society that people with dwarfism enjoy being figures of entertainment. While Alice did not speak out at the time, she now understands why the activist was speaking out against the pantomime. Obviously, for her, the problem is with this kind of show being in town, one minute people are in the theatre laughing at someone with dwarfism, then the next minute they see her and her children going out living life, and people think that it is ok to also laugh at them.

Alice believes that the story of *Snow White and the Seven Dwarfs* should no longer be performed in the pantomime. *Snow White and the Seven Dwarfs* would not be the only show to be cancelled due to controversy. The pantomime performance of the classic tale *Aladdin in Dorset* was cancelled due to 'cultural sensitivities', including names such as 'Chop chop' to refer to Chinese launderette workers (Humphries, 2022). Can we just not tell the story anymore? Can we not just shelve it and say, once upon a time, that was a story read and that people knew, but not anymore? I can remember Disney+ plus [streaming service] back when the Black Lives Matter movement was very popular. Both Disney+ and Netflix [streaming service] made a big statement, saying how they had gone through all of their content to make sure that none of it was seen as racist, and it was not to be shown again. There was a Disney film I used to watch when I was a child, which now that I am older, I realise is now full of racism. Thankfully, it is not on Disney+. Thus, why are we not allowed to say 'Can we stop telling the story of Snow White and the Seven Dwarfs as well' or at least try and change the portrayal of the dwarfs? While entertainment companies, from theatres to streaming services, are removing representations that can be deemed racist, disablist representations have not received the same attention.

Some people think, 'Well, they cannot do these jobs, and they can't do those jobs'. Due to their stature, general society likely considers people with dwarfism to be incapable of working in numerous occupations. Therefore, if general society only sees people with dwarfism as figures of entertainment, as opposed to teachers, lawyers, medics, engineers...,etc. then they are going to believe that the entertainment industry offers them employment.[3] However, most people with dwarfism do not work in the entertainment industry; it is just that it offers more exposure to people with dwarfism. I have made an immense self-discovery that there are no limitations for us. Some of the limitations are what we put there. This can include accepting roles that construct people with dwarfism as figures of fun. The more we keep fighting society and the more we keep showing we can do this, that and everything else, then the more opportunity there is going to be. You do not need to just think oh, *well, that's all I can do*. I would rather be out of work and completely broke before I accept a stag do [Bachelor party] or a hen do [Bachelorette party]. Numerous entertainment companies hire out dwarfs for various celebratory events, such as birthdays and stag dos. Their websites often advertise dwarfs as figures of fun, with limited agency:

> This little guy [dwarf entertainer] can come along, ready to party, and he can handcuff himself to your stag to make sure they aren't parted all day or night...This small bundle of laughs can fit into your itinerary however you want... (Entertain-Ment, 2023)

This example continually emphasises the stature of someone with dwarfism to promote it as a figure of entertainment. Advertising dwarfs for hire demonstrates how the average-sized person hiring the dwarf has complete control over them. In fact, Entertain-Ment's website shows a dwarf handcuffed to a man while at the urinal. I know that money is insane on some of these jobs, but to me, it is still not worth it.[4] It is still not worth not even necessarily what happens to other people with dwarfism and the bullying they then receive. But what could happen to you? You are handcuffed to someone drunk and not in control of what they do. If they suddenly decide they want to jump in a river, you are going with them, and if you cannot swim, well, sorry. It is so dangerous. In 2013, Blake Johnson, a dwarf entertainer who was hired out by St Kilda's football club in Australia, was set on fire by one of the players (ABC News, 2013). In most cases, a dwarf entertainer is

---

[3]For an extensive list of people with dwarfism working in a myriad of occupations, see Adelson, B.M. (2005) *The lives of dwarfs: Their Journey from Public Curiosity Toward Social Liberation*. New Brunswick: Rutgers University Press.

[4]Entertain-Ment's website states that prices start from £150. How much the dwarf entertainer receives from this is not stated.

hired out by a group of people, often inebriated men. The dwarf entertainer has been hired out as a commodity to amuse the party. The reality is that the dwarf entertainer is putting themselves among several men who do not see them as an equal, but rather as a 'plaything' that they can easily overpower. As shown, companies, such as Entertain-Ment, advertise dwarfs for hire in a way that suggests that the person, or group, hiring them out controls the dwarf in any way that is entertaining to them (Pritchard, 2023). In other words, dwarfism is not constructed as a disability, but rather as a novelty that has financial incentives for certain event companies. Thus, if someone with dwarfism wants to change representations of dwarfism, they must avoid any agencies that promote the meta-narrative of dwarfism.

Creating Her Own Destiny

Later Alice left the second agency, to pursue a solo career. Not being part of a casting agency, which specialises in providing short and tall actors, means she is not restricted to roles that focus on her height. Alice is very particular about what kind of work she will do and with whom. Alice regularly has people contacting her, either through her works page or through her social media page on Instagram, often asking if she will fulfil certain roles. Alice considers it important to engage with them to see what the role involves. In one case, she was asked to be a mascot, which she outright refused to do. To be a mascot requires little acting ability, and in this case, Alice was likely wanted purely because of her dwarfism. Writers and producers are likely to have a preconceived idea of dwarfism and the types of acting suitable for them. Therefore, Alice needs to challenge their preconceptions of dwarfism. According to Alice, it is often assumed that people with dwarfism can only fulfil rules, such as the seven dwarfs, which she deems insulting. However, this is not helped by certain dwarf entertainers claiming the removal of these roles robs people with dwarfism of a job (Pritchard, 2023). Alice argues that dwarf entertainers are limiting themselves and insinuating to other people that it is all they can do.

All the things that I was looking for that I thought I would find at places like association for people with dwarfism, I still was not finding it. I was not finding any form of genuine solidarity. I was not finding people on a similar kind of wavelength in terms of thinking; this is outrageous, and this needs to change. Why are we not talking about this? I was not finding anyone that felt the same way. Well, if we keep doing these roles, are we not just perpetuating an ongoing image? If you keep doing the same thing, then people are never going to change their thinking unless you change. They do panto, not because they have a love and a passion for drama and literature. You talk to them about classic plays and you realise they are not actors; they are just suit fillers.

I realised that if I want to get places, I need to have qualifications behind me as well as experience. As a result, I went to a performing Arts college first, and I did my diploma in performing arts, focusing on musical theatre. I would love to see someone with dwarfism being a main character in a musical, such as Evita, or Jesus Christ Superstar. Someone with dwarfism can play those roles, and there does not need to be any kind of joke or pun intended. They can be there because they are good at what they do. The course tutors thought that was a brilliant outlook to have, so that was one of the attributes that luckily got me onto the course.

I got my diploma, and things were going better. I was starting to get more mainstream. I started going for auditions for mainstream roles. It felt amazing to be in a more inclusive environment. I try to avoid roles which specifically request someone with dwarfism unless I know why the producers want someone with dwarfism. I want to show that people with dwarfism are part of everyday society. We all live somewhere, and we are related to people, and we live next to someone, and we drive cars and we have jobs. Therefore, we should be offered roles that reflect everyday life, whether that be in a soap opera or a play. Why do we need to be? 'Oh, and then we have got this character who has got dwarfism, and they do lots of comical things because they are slightly stupid'.

In 2020, the COVID-19 pandemic came along and stopped quite a few of my jobs. Luckily, at this point, I was an Equity member, which was an amazing move to make. Equity is a UK-based, performing arts and entertainment trade union. From my experience, very few people with dwarfism in the industry are not Equity members. As a member of Equity, you have to uphold a certain image. On their website, Equity clearly states that members should be treated with dignity (Equity, 2023). While in 2022, Equity was included within a campaign to target exploitative conditions within the pantomime (Masso, 2022), it does not mean that dwarf actors were necessarily members, especially as some also partake in other forms of dwarf entertainment, which is unlikely to be protected. Some dwarf actors are not members because they want to continue doing derogatory roles. For example, if a person hires themselves out for a stag do and gets hurt, Equity is not going to support them. Firstly, nothing about hiring themselves out is art or performance, and secondly, they should have known the risks before they got into it. So there is not much we can do, whereas Equity protects you. If, say I was to go for a part in something and then I was being bullied or targeted by another cast member or a director, it was evident it was to do with my dwarfism then Equity can stand in. Becoming a member was a brilliant move because it meant I had got that protection.

I joined Equity just before the pandemic, in January 2020. When the pandemic came along, it stopped my work. However, being a member of Equity, I was able to access their benevolent funds. These funds covered work that I had been rehearsing for but was cancelled due to the pandemic. For dwarf entertainers not part of Equity, it would mean that during the pandemic, they would not have been able to partake in dwarf entertainment. For example, due to UK government COVID restrictions, numerous entertainment venues had to cancel performances, including pantomimes. Due to restrictions occurring from March 2020 to December 2021, numerous restrictions meant that celebratory events, such as weddings, had to be cancelled. If some dwarf entertainers rely solely on pantomimes or being hired out, it is unlikely that they would have been able to receive any compensation from their employers.

The pandemic was a life-check moment, where I realised that the entertainment industry can be shut down without any notice or support. As a result, I enroled in a Drama and English degree, as teachers were still able to work. Going to university exposed me to so much more mainstream and so much more to this kind of work that I did modules such as political theatre and experiments in performance. I learnt that these performances were about sending a message out to the audience. These messages could be used to provoke change. It inspired me to think differently about my work.

For the last performance of my degree, I had to completely write my own piece, including the music and staging. My piece was based on height-altering medical procedures, including the new injections – Vosoritide. In 2020, it was announced that there was a new treatment (Vosoritide) for achondroplasia which promises to be a less painful and invasive alternative to limb-lengthening (Saner, 2020). This new treatment has provoked a lot of controversy within the dwarfism community. The treatment is only available to children, and thus, average-sized parents tend to be the main decision-makers. In most cases, parents are opting for the treatment, based on information from the medical industry. While parents try to act in the best interests of their children, people with dwarfism do not always agree with their reasoning. Interventions, including treatments and cures, imply that disabled people cannot be happy or enjoy an adequate quality of life (Swain & French, 2000). People with dwarfism consider these treatments a way of trying to eradicate dwarfism, as the condition is not accepted within society. To highlight this issue, Alice utilises political performance, which engages with some of the sociocultural attitudes that can encourage the use of normalising treatments.

I wanted the performance to portray the lengths that people will go to try and adjust, and adapt their bodies through surgery to feel accepted in society. I managed to get hold of quite a few of the *Vogue* magazines where you have got people with all different disabilities in it. As always, as soon as you have a positive representation, such as a campaign, there is backlash. I will never forget being on social media and reading these comments. One comment stated 'I don't want monsters on my magazine. I just want beautiful people'. Social media is known to engage in disablist hate speech with minimal backlash. Due to poor regulations and promotion of free speech, there are concerns about social media's ability to spread disability hate speech (Burch, 2018; Sherry, 2019). As a response, Alice uses performance to challenge these problematic attitudes and demonstrate her emotional response to them. This type of response means she does not have to engage with internet trolls, but instead an audience that is willing to listen and can leave with more awareness about dwarfism. I used that comment, and the term monsters became a hashtag. In my piece, I am dancing around with the magazine, initially thinking, Oh, my gosh, yes, this is a brilliant representation. Then as I hold the magazine, a phone falls out of it and the music changes. I then pick up and look at the phone, which is projected onto the back screen, with phrases such as 'I don't wanna see monsters, only beautiful people'. After that comes my rage dance, which was my absolute favourite bit. I was wearing this really pretty dress, which I then ripped off, smudged my makeup up my face and started tearing up the magazines. I wanted to emphasise that as soon as we have a great campaign, there is always someone to then shoot it down and make us feel worthless. The performance prompts audiences to be more aware of the attitudes people with dwarfism encounter, their emotional toll upon people with dwarfism and how it can encourage them to undergo normalising medical procedures.

Quite often, normalising procedures are encouraged by family members, which Alice demonstrates in her performance. 'I included the injections and recorded a mock interview between me and my husband, Danny. I said "I don't want to change. I'm happy as I am, it's everyone else that just needs to change their views." I got him to say, "Well, we just want you to be normal and live a normal life, and these injections can help you do that." That interview went on. Then I went up to this table that I prepared with these massive syringes filled with baby moisturiser. I had to colour it red because I wanted a bold colour that stood out. The scene just involved me injecting myself. I then began to change my physical appearance to being, where I had managed to just dance around on the stage. Now, I am struggling to even stand, because, as is the issue with any type of procedure, there is always a risk factor'. Historical treatments for dwarfism often result in numerous complications and in some cases fatalities (Pritchard, 2023). I remember watching a documentary about heightism. There was a lady who had over lengthened her arms and legs, and she could barely walk.[5] The aim was to highlight that you should have just left alone. The moisturiser is dripping off of me and I used my dad's old walking frame to support myself and make myself seem unable to move properly again, and then I just use the line 'Am I still a monster now?' The idea was that I was trying to change to fit in. I had made myself worse and more disabled by trying to change my disability. I am pleased to say there was not a dry eye in the house. That is not to say I like to make people cry, but it means they got the message. Kuppers (2004) suggests that disabled artists use performance as a way to express themselves and as a form of activism. Performance art helps to express the artist's message to a wide range of people. In this case, treatments are not always for the better. One of the biggest divides between parents and people with dwarfism is the result of conflicting attitudes concerning treatments for people with dwarfism (Pritchard, 2023). Through performance, Alice can express her concerns about these treatments, which could help to inform parents of children with dwarfism.

Conclusion

Alice's experiences of performing in the pantomime challenge the notion that is suitable work for people with dwarfism. It uncovers how performing as one of Snow White's seven dwarfs is not as appropriate as made to be in society. Alice's experiences expose the emotional toll performing as one of the seven dwarfs had on her, which general society is unaware of. The seven dwarfs, albeit Grumpy, are

---

[5]This would have been as a result of limb-lengthening, a procedure which involves surgery to break both legs (and sometimes arms) then having them set with screws which are turned each day for several months in order to encourage new bone to grow in between, thus lengthening the limbs. Limb-lengthening is described as having 'high complication rate and significant morbidity with a relatively long period of disability during the process even when no complications occur' (Moseley, 1989, p. 38).

framed as cheerful characters. This coupled with the longevity of the show encourages people to believe that dwarfs are happy to be in the pantomime.

Agencies specifically for people with dwarfism often reinforce stereotypical roles for dwarfs, which in this chapter, Alice refers to as 'suit fillers'. Even worse, there are now a growing number of event agencies that hire out dwarfs as 'party novelties'. This chapter shows that it is still possible for people with dwarfism to be successful, without having to rely on agencies and companies which profit from derogatory representations of dwarfism.

This chapter has shown that internalised ableism held by many dwarf entertainers impacts the voices of others striving for equality. This demonstrates that the quest for more positive representations of dwarfism is not only hindered by average-sized writers and producers but also dwarf performers. Furthermore, the UK-based association for people with dwarfism [association for people with dwarfism] seems to encourage people with dwarfism to pursue stereotypical roles associated with dwarfism.

Alice has demonstrated how gaining an education and being a member of a trade union has enabled her to challenge stereotypes of dwarfism. Using performance art, Alice can highlight contemporary political issues impacting people with dwarfism, such as the push for height-altering treatments.

References

ABC News. (2013). Dwarf entertainer allegedly set on fire in St Kilda 'Mad Monday' event [online]. https://www.abc.net.au/news/2013-09-03/dwarf-entertainer-allegedly-set-on-fire-in-st-kilda-27mad-mond/4930858?nw=0. Accessed on September 29, 2023.
Bogdan, R. (1988). *Freak show: Presenting human oddities for amusement and profit.* University of Chicago Press.
Burch, L. (2018). 'You are a parasite on the productive classes': Online disablist hate speech in austere times. *Disability & Society*, *33*(3), 392–415.
Entertain-Ment. (2023). Stag do dwarf hire. [online]. https://www.entertain-ment.co.uk/stag-party-ideas/dwarf-hire-stag-do. Accessed on September 28, 2023.
Equity. (2023). Dignity at work. https://www.equity.org.uk/advice-and-support/know-your-rights/right-to-equal-treatment/disability. Accessed on September 27, 2023.
Humphries, W. (2022). Magic is over for 'culturally insensitive' Aladdin. *The Times* [online]. https://www.thetimes.co.uk/article/magic-is-over-for-culturally-insensitive-aladdin-xc2lfm888#:~:text=A%20pantomime%20production%20of%20Aladdin,before%20the%20decision%20was%20made. Accessed on September 28, 2023.
Ktenidis, A. (2022). En/counters with disablist school violence: Experiences of young people with dwarfism in the United Kingdom. *British Journal of Sociology of Education*, *43*(8), 1196–1215.
Kuppers, P. (2004). *Disability and contemporary performance: Bodies on edge.* Routledge.
Masso, G. (2022). 'Exploitative' pantomime conditions targeted by campaign. *The Stage* [online]. https://www.thestage.co.uk/news/exploitative-pantomime-conditions-targeted-by-campaign. Accessed on September 29, 2023.

Moseley, C. F. (1989). Leg lengthening: A review of 30 years. *Clinical Orthopaedics and Related Research®*, *247*, 38–43.

Pritchard, E. (2023). *Midgetism: The exploitation and discrimination of people with dwarfism*. Routledge.

Pritchard, E. (2022). "Get down on your knees": Representing the seven dwarfs in the pantomime. *Disability Studies Quarterly*, *42*(1).

Saner, E. (2020). 'There is a fear that this will eradicate dwarfism': The controversy over a new growth drug. *The Guardian* [online]. https://www.theguardian.com/science/2020/sep/28/there-is-a-fear-that-this-will-eradicate-dwarfism-the-controversy-over-a-new-growth-drug. Accessed on September 28, 2023.

Sherry, M. (2019). Disablist hate speech online. In M. Sherry, T. Olsen, J. Vedeler, & J. Eriksen (Eds.), *Disability hate speech: Social, cultural and political contexts* (pp. 40–66). Routledge.

Sladen, S. (2017). 'Hiya fans!': Celebrity performance and reception in modern British Pantomime. In A. Ainsworth, O. Double, & L. Peacock (Eds.), *Popular performance* (pp. 179–202). Bloomsbury.

Swain, J., & French, S. (2000). Towards an affirmation model of disability. *Disability & Society*, *15*(4), 569–582.

Watson, K. (2020). "With a smile and a song": Representations of people with dwarfism in 1930s cinema. *Journal of Literary & Cultural Disability Studies*, *14*(2), 137–153.

Chapter 5

Midgitte Bardot: Using Drag Performance to Challenge People's Perceptions and Attitudes of Dwarfism

Tamm Reynolds (Drag Artist)
UK

Erin Pritchard (Senior Lecturer in Disability Studies)
Liverpool Hope University, UK

Introduction

Midgitte Bardot is Tamm Reynolds' drag alter ego, who they have been performing as, in various UK venues since 2017. While drag performances are well known for expressing queer identity, in this chapter Tamm Reynolds reflects upon how engaging in drag performances allows them to push for a more positive and realistic dwarf identity. Drag shows have a history of combining politics with entertainment (Taylor et al., 2004). This intersection between sexuality and disability, both of which have been oppressed throughout history, permits Tamm to engage with political performances. Tamm, who can be considered a crip, queer solo performer, believes that having a drag alter ego permits them to do anything with an air of confidence that someone like them is usually not afforded. In this case, it is to be sexy, while exposing the everyday discrimination they face as a person with dwarfism. This is not only to raise awareness but also to challenge any preconceived ideas that the audience may have about dwarfism.

This chapter explores how Midgitte's performances often include shocking material, which some may find offensive. In particular, Tamm includes a poem they recites to audiences to express the psycho-emotional disablism she faces as a result of the actions of one midget entertainer. However, this poem is not the usual offence that you would expect. Instead of mocking people with dwarfism, it mocks a midget entertainer to demonstrate the anger they feel towards them due to the repercussions people like her experience as a result of the choices they make. Referring to themselves as a 'political freak', Tamm demonstrates how they engages in shock performance to raise awareness.

Dwarfism Arts and Advocacy, 63–74
Copyright © 2024 Tamm Reynolds and Erin Pritchard
Published under exclusive licence by Emerald Publishing Limited
doi:10.1108/978-1-83753-922-220241011

Introducing Midgitte Bardot

Midgitte's performances are an intersection of LGBTQIA+ and disability, engaging with both queer and crip work. One of their latest appearances was in the 2023 July edition of the iconic fashion magazine Vogue, in the LGBTQIA+ special issue of the magazine. Engaging with drag, the purpose of Midgitte Bardot is to provide a queer crip solo performance that challenges the audience's expectations of dwarfism and to change their perspective and attitudes about the condition. Performers who identify as both crip and queer in their work provide us with not only a verbal articulation of these issues but with 'an embodied text' (Sandahl, 2003, p. 25). As a result, Tamm refers to themselves as a 'political freak'. A political freak can be described as a performer whose identity differs from the norm, such as a drag artist or a disabled person, to challenge beliefs and change perceptions about them. Midgitte's performances involve entering the stage and doing everything in her own time. I think what I try to do is subvert an expectation every time there is one. When I come on stage I get in a cabaret setting. Normally people would come on stage, be full of energy and interact with the audience. However, I will probably come on 10 or 15 seconds after my name's been called. I will put my drink down somewhere on the stage. I will see if the props are there. I will arrange my wig and probably will not look at the audience yet. I am just not interested in what they have got to offer yet. Maybe I will wait for them to finish cheering me. I might talk into the mic and say, 'Hi! Firstly, I'll sing a song for you, but before that song, I'm going to say a few words, and then we will go home afterwards'. I think, because dwarfism is so mystified, I really enjoy whenever there is a smoke and mirrors opportunity. I will blow the smoke away and I will show you the mirror. I very much enjoy that as a performer. I think that creates a sense of unease.

I do my classic job of doing a kind of talking spiel. I am quite funny and comedic. I have got a great sense of timing. I think I have learnt a sense of timing, but I think I was born with a sense of timing. I was also born with dwarfism, and I do think that there is probably a connection going on there. In some ways, I am not saying it is inherent, but again, there is a hypervigilance that happens where you become extremely aware, and you learn about people really fast. So, you can kind of see how someone will laugh.

Midgitte does not care about how people around her are reacting to her body or how she interacts with a man-made environment built for someone much taller than her. This is why sometimes when Midgitte comes on stage she will take her time to get on a chair that is too high for her. I want them to be more acutely aware of the space in between us like we are. I want them to feel too big for the place. I want them to feel extremely privileged to experience this world in the way they do. That is what I am trying to generate and play with, and I want to do that with visuals and by changing the shape of the space and the seats that they sit in being able to demonstrate that we have had different lives, and will always lead different experiences because of the world that has been made by them. When a person with dwarfism interacts with a space differently, due to a mismatch in height between them and the space, it can result in unwanted attention from other people (Pritchard, 2021a). As a form of deflection, Tamm believes that the extravagant clothing and make-up that they adorn to become Midgitte Bardot takes some of the focus from their dwarf body and instead places the audience's gaze upon the appearance they have chosen. Therefore interacting with a space differently, while dressed as Midgitte, deflects attention from Tamm.

Midgitte Bardot is a drag alter ego performance persona that I created back in 2017 which is when I started doing drag. Before that, I was hosting and performing in open mic nights. But I started getting into the idea of the disruption that my body can cause and create. I quite enjoyed experimenting with drag as a medium to do that with. I also enjoyed it and it felt safer to create an alter ego, which then meant that I could do things I would not normally do and say things I would not normally say, but if I was Midgitte Bardot, then I would feel quite safe to do that. Midgitte provides a different persona to Tamm, which offers her the opportunity to express herself in a way that she would not feel as confident doing as Tamm. To aid in deflecting attention from Tamm, Midgitte dons eye-catching costumes, which aid in deflecting attention from her body. I have only recently been able to interrogate what happens to me on stage as Midgitte. I very much feel like a bit of a vessel, a different embodiment. I noticed that one of Midgitte's traits, which is probably a bit more intentional, is that she is very cool, very calm and very collected. Having that as part of her persona, I would say, has been a coping mechanism to the stressful and taxing experience of being a performer with a non-normative body. I feel safe performing as Midgitte Bardot because I think there is an element where, when I am in drag, I am already demanding or there is some kind of social contract where it is saying you can look at me now. I am telling you to look at me so when I have done that as just, and also being called Midgitte immediately.

The name Midgitte Bardot plays homage to the French actress Bridgitte Bardot. Automatically, Tamm challenges the notion that people with dwarfism are asexual (Pritchard, 2021b), by adopting an alter ego that is based on an actress regarded as a sex symbol. Rearticulating labels that society has used to disempower and humiliate minority groups, in this case, people with dwarfism, can be empowering (Sandahl, 2003). Midgitte Bardot is a Drag Cabaret performer, who is sexy and will often dress in skimpy clothing, showing off her cleavage ('tits are a big part of Midgitte's personality!') demonstrating how someone with dwarfism can be sexual. 'A primary way for crip queer solo performers to express disability pride is to rearticulate the disabled body as a gendered, sexual being' (Sandahl, 2003, p. 44). Tamm states, 'If you are going to look, then I am going to look fantastic'. Drag performances are known to disrupt typical understandings of sexuality (Taylor et al., 2004). In this case, drag is used to make a body that is usually deemed asexual, sexual.

What Midgitte wears is an important part of her performance, which challenges preconceived ideas about dwarfism, including the notion that dwarfs are asexual. Being sexual is a big part of Midgitte's personality. She is very sexual. She does not necessarily perform in a sexualised way, but she wears sexy clothing, such as netted fish nets with big holes in them, big boots, some kind of tight dress, a big wig and a push-up Bra which gives her big tits. That has been her look for as long as I can remember. 'Unlike able-bodied women whose bodies are over-determined sexually, disabled performers struggle to be considered sexual beings at all and tend to use nudity and provocative clothing simply to claim a sexual identity' (Sandahl, 2003, p. 45).

Midgitte's outfits provide a juxtaposition between the ability for someone with a non-normative body to be sexy and conceive themselves as such. I think Miss Piggy is a very big inspiration for Midgitte. I enjoy just the way that she looks, and I think she is beautiful, and I love her personality, born and dying diva, and she ought to be like that for the rest of her life as she should be, and we should all be listening to that. There is also this element of the joke of Miss Piggy that she is a pig and she is the most beautiful woman in the world. I think Midgitte is similar; she is a force to be reckoned with and feels very much in control. She is slow, she takes her time, and she is also really sexy, she knows it, and she's a dwarf.

The Adoption of Queer Spaces

Both disabled people and members of LGBTQIA+ have experienced marginalisation, which has often led them to occupy particular spaces. I perform in mostly queer places, but also bars, venues, theatres and live art spaces. Going out in queer spaces, I would experience active protection via the means of drag queens who were working on the door, which meant that I always felt quite safe in those spaces. When you are a performer in those spaces, you are not only safe, but you are also royalty. The acceptance of a dwarf body within these spaces can be down to the fact that both disabled people and members of LGBTQIA+ share a history of marginalisation and injustice. It makes sense that the people who experience some of the most intense marginalisation and abuse outside of those walls are the ones who want to go into them and perform as royalty, and feel safe there. However, Tamm states that queer spaces need to be more accessible for disabled people. Thus, while the meaning of a space can make it inclusive, for disabled people to access these spaces, they must also be physically accessible.

I could have joined an acting group. I could have gone into drama and more theatre route and been cast with people with dwarfism. That is the road I could have gone down, but instead, I went down the punk transgressive, queer road. There is something that I do not relate to with disability art, which I think is a degree of earnestness, perhaps, or sincerity. I think I have that in my own work, anyway. I feel that dwarfism is still not recognised by a lot of other disabled people as a disability. I have had quite a few very disappointing interactions in that world, which made me feel as excluded as I already do in most other areas. I remember one person said to me, 'Do you identify as disabled?' And I said, 'Yes, I do'. And they said, 'Oh, how?' And I said 'dwarfism!' And then they said, 'Did you say autism?' And I said 'No, dwarfism'. And then they said, 'Oh, I didn't think dwarfism was a disability'. This was disability arts. It was very strange. But I think again, this is what is tricky, is that I do not like saying disability art, because that is one person. There are multiple others.

Dwarfism is often contested as a disability. An influential factor in dwarfism's contention as a disability is its historical representations, such as being constructed as 'freakish' (Ablon, 1990; Kruse, 2003). Even in the present day, there are representations of dwarfism that exist, such as midget tossing, that would be less tolerated if associated with other disabled people. Hence, why Tamm recognises that dwarfism does not resonate fully with other disabled people, including within the arts. Tamm recognises that representations of dwarfism differ and subsequently identifies themselves more closely with other minority groups, including those who identify as fat.

There is something about dwarfism that feels a bit like it sits in between disability and something else, and I am not entirely sure what that is. I do not know if it is just plain old prejudice, or being a 'freak of culture'. That is something that resonates with me. It is something that I have always kind of thought about especially when I am in mostly disability circles. That kind of chat about being a freak in the way the media essentially portrays you. That is not something that all disabled people can relate to and there are also a lot of people who are not disabled who do relate to that, including people who identify as Fat. There is a very common crossover of similar treatment, and similar humiliation attempts and techniques and this act of humiliation and ridicule that we experience is a lot more interesting to me as an artist and a performer. I would rather go to places where those are intersecting and crossing over in terms of the identity of the people who I would be performing alongside or in the venues that I would be in. I guess I do not feel like I have been seen really in the disability arts world. I feel more seen in basements, clubs, queer drag bars and live art spaces.

Using Drag to Challenge Midgetism

As a performer, I was always thinking about what the audience would be expecting from a dwarf performer called Midgitte Bardot, who does drag. Midgitte is of course a play on the word 'midget'. A term, which Tamm knows is problematic, but as an artist, they constantly push the boundaries of what is normal and what is expected within society. Tamm argues that by reclaiming the term midget, the person who is the object of the joke, takes back the term and is thus in control. In other words, they have used it before anyone else can, and in a way that empowers them. Drag performances are known for their contestation, to subvert dominant power relations (Taylor et al., 2004). It is very disarming and a reversal of power. They also purposely include a word associated with dwarfism, even in a negative way, for the audience to be aware that the performer has dwarfism before they come on stage. Midgitte gives off the energy of 'I already know what you are thinking, or wanting to think or what you're trying not to think' and so I feel I am in a position of power as Midgitte. It also means that they will listen to me, but at the same time take me a bit less seriously because of the drag, which sometimes is great and sometimes is annoying. I quite enjoy being able to feel a bit freer to express myself. There is a clear line of you are talking to Midgitte.

People with dwarfism often have to anticipate the presence of new people. How will they react to someone with dwarfism? Will they laugh and snigger? Will they feel uncomfortable? Thus, Tamm believes that by having a drag name that denotes that she has dwarfism will remove any unwanted reactions of surprise. People with dwarfism often feel anxious when venturing out in public as they anticipate the unwanted reactions, such as staring, pointing and laughter from others, which are commonplace in their daily lives.

I think when I first started performing, I realised that there is a unanimous lived experience, specifically for people with dwarfism where the thought that goes through your head when you're about to meet a new group of people or a new person, or anything like that, or walk into a room that you have not walked into before, and these people are going to be expecting me. I need to pre-empt how they are going to react. I always think about that and it creates this sense of hypervigilance. Tamm uses drag to remove those anxieties and to alter audiences' perceptions of their dwarf body. Tamm wants to repurpose and reclaim that word. As Midgitte, she wants to own the word to rid the Elephant in the room. However, are they then expecting a midget entertainer? Someone who engages with slapstick for the audience to laugh at.[1]

Tamm Reynold's does not pander to anyone, including people with dwarfism. As she previously stated 'I am very aware that people with dwarfism might hate me because my name is Midgitte Bardot. I think it makes people uncomfortable' (Magill, 2020). The play on the term midget is their attempt at reclaiming it. Using the term is a reversal of power, but ensuring it is not used in a derogatory manner can only be done through ensuring that their actual performances challenge what is usually expected from a performer with dwarfism. Tamm believes that their drag alter ego needs to be radical, and to do this she utilises queer spaces, including clubs, basements, as well as live art clubs and theatres. They believes that these spaces, which historically have been stigmatised, are more accepting of the dwarf body than typical, normate spaces (Pritchard, 2023). According to Chappell (2015), both disabled people and the LGBTQIA+ community share a similar history of social injustice, oppression and isolation as they challenge hegemonic constructs of normalcy. Tamm demonstrates how the spaces they occupy as a drag performer has made them feel accepted. Drag performances are known for promoting solidarity and staging political resistance (Taylor et al., 2004). Drag is something that gives them confidence and a sense of belonging. It reverses the power relations, between them and the audience, who are predominantly non-disabled and of average stature. It is something she believes she can get attention safely, but recognises that in the current political climate, drag is not safe. In the United States drag performances are being banned, including in the state of Tennessee, as they are considered devious and dangerous by some people (Nossel, 2023). Yet, these same states will unapologetically hold midget tossing or

---

[1]Midget is not used as a slur, but as an academic term to identify those who partake in entertainment that reinforces problematic stereotypes of dwarfism. These representations often solely focus on the entertainer's height, which is constructed in a derogatory manner, such as being a figure of fun.

midget wrestling events.[2] This makes them question how society readily accepts midget entertainment, but frowns upon drag, especially when drag performers interact with children.

Tamm believes that the pantomime is more traumatic and damaging for children, especially for children with dwarfism than drag is. Imagine, being a child with dwarfism and seeing somebody who shares your condition being humiliated on stage. Imagine being surrounded by an audience who are pointing and laughing at 'the dwarfs', which makes you anxious about getting up from your seat when the show finally ends. As a result, Tamm provides a performance that does not adhere to midget entertainment.

I think it is quite exciting to be me, just as Tamm and as Midgitte, loving attention and loving, performing and being good at it and having a presence. There is also another element where I am going to try to offer something that they have not seen before. If there is another person of dwarfism in the room then that is great. They can watch something that I have chosen and wanted to do and it has shaken the room a little bit at the same time, which is wonderful. That is not an experience we, as people with dwarfism, get very often. The experience we get normally is of someone with dwarfism doing a performance that they probably did not sign up for, did not really want to do, but were told to do. The room has probably been more excited about this, and we have been the ones who have been shaken, and think that it was horrible, yet everyone loved it. It is rather put on us. Of course, midget entertainers have free choice in taking those roles, but Tamm does not believe any child with dwarfism grows up wanting to dress as an Oompa Loompa or wants to hire themselves out.

Midgitte is a character that is constructed to avoid oppressing people with dwarfism. Drag performances are known for communicating counter identification to reject or mock gender stereotypes (Taylor et al., 2004). Similarly, Midgitte uses drag performance to reject cultural stereotypes associated with dwarfism, but with a slight nod to it. In one performance Midgitte wears an ill-fitting Oompa Loompa costume that she slowly takes off and discards, to show that while the audience may expect dwarfs to dress up like this, most of us have complete disregard for it. Again, Midgitte uses a particular costume to challenge preconceived ideas about dwarfism.

Tamm reflects upon some of the choices midget entertainers make, and reflects upon how they would want their younger self to feel watching that exact performance. Midgitte Bardot's performances are known for criticising midget entertainment. She wants to hold midget entertainers accountable for their actions. These actions play into the social oppression people with dwarfism experience and as a result impact the psycho-emotional well-being of people with dwarfism, which Thomas (2007) refers to as psycho-emotional disablism.

---

[2]Tamm adopts Pritchard's (2023) reclaiming and repurposing of the word 'midget' to refer to entertainment that engages with 'midgetism', in other words entertainment that reinforces problematic beliefs about dwarfism.

When I see people who have my body, doing jobs or gigs, or work, or performing in kind of roles that seem to be dehumanising them, whether that is a goblin or a fantastical dwarf of another time, or a leprechaun, it has had a knock-on effect on my self-esteem regarding what I thought my body and my job prospects in the future could be, or would be. Growing up as a child with dwarfism and as an adult with dwarfism there are a lot of extremely difficult problems, and we face lots of different challenges, but one of them that I think, has a deeper knock-on effect is the cultural stereotypes and connotations and representations of dwarfism in mainstream, very accessible media.

I perform a lot of monologues to think about different power dynamics. One monologue is about the career path of Warwick Davis, who due to some of the roles he has chosen can place him as a midget entertainer.[3] Warwick has been in some Hollywood blockbusters, such as Star Wars and Harry Potter. Numerous roles Warwick has undertaken are what Alice Lambert refers to in Chapter 4 as 'suit filler' roles. For example, in Star Wars he played an Ewok and in numerous Harry Potter films, he played one of the Goblins of Gringotts Wizarding Bank. A lot of things he has done are very mythical, or use prosthetics and plays into the carnival freak show, the monstrous fantastical, such as goblins and leprechauns. My work is often about challenging him on his career path and his choices in the roles, and then parallelling it with my experiences of dwarfism.

Hollywood feels like the world, and it felt like I was being told to look at Warwick's body like it is this 'freakish thing', too. It is quite confusing for a child and can inspire shame and internalised midgetism, and I think probably isolated me. I thought I was supposed to find Warwick to be a role model but he represents things that are used to make fun of me. I believe that as a dwarf performer, where you are sharing yourself with the world, you have to hold yourself responsible for the effects it is going to have on the people in your community who are being called lots of different names. Outside of all of those fantastical roles he worked with Ricky Gervais on *Life's Too Short* (2011–2013) which then made another opportunity for adults this time to feel okay about making fun of people with dwarfism because they have done it on television. For example, Warwick Davis is famous, which makes it acceptable and that was extremely annoying.

Tamm recites a poem as Midgitte Bardot for Warwick. The aim of the poem is to the negative impact of his work upon people with dwarfism including Tamm.

> You... have made my life harder.
> You don't know me - but you have made my life harder.
> The body I have is ridiculed because of the body you have and how you have used it. How you have let others use it and use you. So publicly. You have told people it's okay to laugh at difference, at

---

[3] A person with dwarfism who chooses to partake in entertainment which reinforces midgetism (Pritchard, 2023).

deformity - at me.
I have lost agency over my body and the space around it because of choices you have made. I don't even know you.
People tell me to look to you for inspiration. Those people don't understand the damage you've done and the damage you keep doing to society's perception of me. Now I am always public because people have seen you, doing what you do and they laughed at you. They're not laughing with you, Warwick, it's at you. And now... it's at me.

You've made your body about your height, you microscopic malarial mosquito. Your white-cis-male-straight-rich body. And, so, my body is now about how it stands next to yours, or Verne's [Verne Troyer]. Your body in those fantasy flicks, yours in that sitcom about the perils of fame, of being an arsehole. I'm not a fantasy and I'm not famous and I'm not always an arsehole.

My body is not about my height – though I am very, very short - it's about the circus-freak-culture that your illustrious career has contributed to oh-so-generously. But, Warwick - I would hate to disregard your oh-so-philanthropic Dwarf acting agency and how it has paved the way towards the midget-Macbeth we are all asking for. But alas! Poor Warwick...
oh shit that's Hamlet, isn't it?

You do PANTO [pantomime], for fucks sake. The first time I saw another dwarf was in Snow White and that made me think that's the only place I was good for – to serve as a minor gag in a pretty white ladies' rom-com.

You're the reason I had leg lengthening operations both when I was seven and again when I was fourteen and I was supposed to have it when I was 11 but I got too scared in the anaesthetic room and backed out but it was okay because my consultant said she could have an early lunch break so that means it wasn't a big deal and my crippling yes crippling doubt about changing myself and my body and being in pain for months and months on end so that I could fit into the world that wasn't built for me was fine because my long long long long long LOOONNG legged doctor got to have her tuna mayo sandwich sooner than she anticipated and–
I had those operations because I was born into a world that doesn't accept my body and you did nothing but fuel that notion.

I was a wheelchair-user. And you know what? I experienced less shit, than I do by just being a dwarf. Good job, Warwick, keep up the hard work.

This is not the full poem, but a few extracts that Tamm recites as Midgitte Bardot. Tamm explained to me how as a performer they push the boundaries and can often go too far. Hence why they refer to themselves as a 'political freak', someone who uses drag performance to challenge people's disablist ideas. The poem demonstrates how Tamm is robbed of agency, and the psycho-emotional impact Warwick's performances have upon them. Tamm holds Warwick Davis, as well as other midget entertainers to account by revealing the repercussions their choices have upon other people with dwarfism. Tamm emphasises that the choices that Warwick makes, result in society's perception of them.

Midget entertainers such as Warwick are some people's only point of reference to dwarfism and thus people believe that how they permit themselves to be perceived and treated by audiences is how other people with dwarfism can be. Drag show audiences have reported that the shows make them stop and think about typical stereotypes associated with LGBTQIA+ minorities, often changing their perceptions for the better (Taylor et al., 2004). I want the audience to leave feeling a bit enlightened about harmful stereotypes of people dwarfism and how it affects us, the damage and hurt to our self-esteem, confidence, our safety, our job prospects and our rights.

Tamm anticipates that outside of the dwarfism community, Warwick is held in high regard. For example, the Shaw Trust often includes Warwick Davis in its annual list of the 100 most influential disabled people in the United Kingdom. According to the Shaw Trust, the aim of the list is to 'To bring together the most influential disabled people in Britain and shine a light on their successes. Encouraging the talented leaders of tomorrow to connect with role models and see that aspiration and ambition can be fulfiled regardless of disability or impairment' (De Havilland, 2021, n.d.). However, for people with dwarfism, those who partake in midget entertainment, such as pantomimes, are not always deemed good role models. For years people with dwarfism have been turning their back on the entertainment industry (Adelson, 2005), especially as they realise the impact midget entertainment has on their social standing. However, this change does not seem to have registered within the wider society. The Shaw Trust claims that it wants to change the public's perception of disability, but it will not change the public's perception of dwarfism by holding a person who reinforces midgetism, in such high regard.

The poem offers Tamm's audience a new perspective, one that is informed by the emotional impact midget entertainment has upon them. Of course, Warwick is not the only midget entertainer to influence how she as well as other people with dwarfism are perceived and treated within society. While Midgitte also mentions the late midget entertainer Verne Troyer, Warwick is used as a reference to all midget entertainers. However, using him, probably the most well known, British midget entertainer, makes the audiences rethink their perceptions of him and what he does. Perhaps the Shaw Trust should listen?

A powerful part of Tamm's poem is the insight as to why she underwent leg-lengthening as a child, which as shown is a very long drawn out and painful procedure. Yet, this is something they felt they needed to do to fit into society. They attempted to change their body to not be associated with the notion of dwarfism that people like Warwick encourage. That is a big commitment to make and shows how much of a negative impact midget entertainment has on people with dwarfism and how much they want to be disassociated with it.

Conclusion

Performing as Midgitte Bardot permits Tamm to challenge ableist stereotypes. Drag is another way for artists with dwarfism to create their own identity and push back at the one that is often placed upon them. Performing as Midgitte allows Tamm to be sexual. This chapter has shown how drag performances that intersect with disability can aid in challenging hegemonic beliefs about dwarfism.

As Midgitte, performing in spaces she feels more comfortable within allows Tamm to raise awareness about dwarfism. This chapter has shown that the spaces she performs in are important in providing the right power dynamics that come from feeling accepted.

This chapter has questioned how midget entertainment is readily accepted by society, despite its damage to people with dwarfism. Tamm shows, through their alter ego Midgitte Bardot, the problems of midget entertainment, including its emotional impact upon those who do not partake in it, but nonetheless experience its unwanted repercussions.

References

Ablon, J. (1990). Ambiguity and difference: Families with dwarf children. *Social Science and Medicine, 30*(8), 879–887.

Adelson, B. (2005). The changing lives of archetypal 'curiosities' – And echoes of the past. *Disability Studies Quarterly, 25*(3), 1–13.

Chappell, P. (2015). Queering the social emergence of disabled sexual identities: Linking queer theory with disability studies in the South African context. *Agenda, 29*(1), 54–62.

De Havilland, A. (2021). The power of the disability power 100. *The Shaw Trust* [online]. https://disabilitypower100.com/?s=warwick+davis. Accessed on September 28, 2023.

Kruse, R. (2003). Narrating intersections of gender and dwarfism in everyday spaces. *Canadian Geographer, 47*(4), 494–508.

Magill, J. (2020). "I can't get deep in the way I want to": Killing Midgitte Bardot and becoming Tam Reynolds. *The State of the Arts* [online]. https://www.thestateofthearts.co.uk/features/i-cant-get-deep-in-the-way-i-want-to-get-deep-killing-midgitte-bardot-and-becoming-tammy-reynolds/. Accessed on July 25, 2023.

Nossel, S. (2023). The drag show bans sweeping the US are a chilling attack on free speech. *The Guardian* [online]. https://www.theguardian.com/culture/commentisfree/2023/mar/10/drag-show-bans-tennessee-lgbtq-rights. Accessed on July 25, 2023.

Pritchard, E. (2021a). *Dwarfism, spatiality and disabling experiences.* Routledge.

Pritchard, E. (2021b). The metanarrative of dwarfism: Heightism and its social implications. In D. Bolt (Ed.), *The metanarrative of disability: Culture, assumed authority, and the normative social order* (pp. 123–137). Routledge.

Pritchard, E. (2023). *Midgetism: The exploitation and discrimination of people with dwarfism.* Routledge.

Sandahl, C. (2003). Queering the crip or cripping the queer?: Intersections of queer and crip identities in solo autobiographical performance. *GLQ: A Journal of Lesbian and Gay Studies*, 9(1), 25–56.

Taylor, V., Rupp, L. J., & Gamson, J. (2004). Performing protest: Drag shows as tactical repertoire of the gay and lesbian movement. In D. Myers & D. Cress (Eds.), *Authority in contention* (pp. 105–137). Emerald Publishing Limited.

Thomas, C. (2007). *Sociologies of disability and illness: Contested ideas in disability Studies and medical sociology.* Palgrave Macmillan.

Chapter 6

The Path to Success Is Long and Winding: Challenging Stereotypes and Fighting for Disability Equality in the Entertainment Industry

Danny Woodburn (Actor and Disability Activist)
USA

Erin Pritchard (Senior Lecturer in Disability Studies)
Liverpool Hope University, UK

Introduction

Danny Woodburn has been acting since he graduated from Temple University, majoring in Film and Theatre, in 1989. He is probably most well known for playing Mickey Abbott in the popular television show, Seinfeld (1989–1998). However, Danny has also starred in numerous other films and television shows, all of which he ensures do not reinforce problematic stereotypes of dwarfism. According to Adelson (2005, p. 283) 'Woodburn has noted that he is selective and at times turns down dehumanising roles, even when doing so results in unemployment, but that as a fortunate result, he is offered bigger and better parts, which are not specifically written for little people'.

In 2001, Danny received an Outstanding Alumni Achievement Award. While actors with dwarfism, including Danny, have been rightly celebrated and admired for refusing roles which perpetuate ableist stereotypes, there has been limited acknowledgement of the backlash these actors have received from writers and producers. In a study consisting of disabled actors from the Screen Actors Guild (SAG), Raynor and Hayward (2009) identified several barriers to employment including industry attitudes about working with disabled actors, actors being restricted to specific roles and fears about requesting accommodations. In this chapter, Danny Woodburn explores all of these issues.

Danny converses about how he has had to negotiate with writers and producers who have often resorted to engaging with problematic stereotypes of dwarfism in their productions. These negotiations demonstrate unequal power relations that make ableism difficult to challenge. While some have been open to suggested changes from Danny, others have resulted in conflicts and lost employment opportunities for him. This chapter demonstrates the difficulties involved in the push for more realistic roles that do not engage with harmful stereotypes of dwarfism.

Another conflict of interest is issues of access, which can make it difficult for disabled actors to make it as what Danny terms 'elite actors'. He is not just an actor, but also an advocate for disabled people in the entertainment industry. Access issues can hinder opportunities. In this chapter, Danny explains the importance of access and providing disabled actors with more opportunities which can further their careers. A good example is Danny's 'Woodburn ratio', a tool for dealing with the controversial practice of cripping up. He demonstrates how a lack of access for disabled actors enables excuses for performances that engage with cripping up.

How It All Started

Going back to the love of performance, it stems from the desire to entertain my mother and brothers. When I was four-years old I used to improvise to an old 78 speed Woody Guthrie Album called *Songs to Grow On*. A 78 Speed is sort of an obsolete, odd-shaped record. I do not know why we had this record, but I used to act out the songs as a child and try to make people laugh.

I think, for the longest time, I wanted to be a veterinarian. I loved animals, and we always had cats and dogs in the house. So I pursued science through high school, although I took one drama class. I never auditioned for any plays in high school. However, Danny's aim to pursue a career in Veterinary Science was impacted by his need for multiple surgeries.

Right after high school, I had to have my third round of osteotomies on my hips, knees and ankles. I had my knees done as a kid. Each knee was done as a boy of five, and then I had both hips done where I was in a full hip spica cast, and body cast, I had both hips done when I was 12-years old. When I was 18 I was scheduled to do it again, so I had to put college on hold. But then, my doctor, who was sort of the patron saint of little people when it comes to orthopaedics, had to postpone; his wife's mother passed away. It was postponed for about six months.

I started to take a couple of classes at my local college, but I had to drop out because of a spontaneous detached retina, which is another part of my syndrome. After that surgery healed, I finally went to go see him. That surgery probably shut me down for eight or nine months of my life. I was in a cast for four and a half months and then had to have 6–8 weeks of physical therapy. A good portion of that was in a hospital.

In these instances, Danny's education was impacted by secondary conditions associated with dwarfism. As a result, he began to take classes in the arts. During that time I had a lot of time to consider where I wanted to go and what I wanted to do with my life. I got interested in film school, especially in acting and performing. I started at Temple University, in what they called radio television and film and then I switched to a theatre major after the first semester, and then I switched back to radio television and film after the next semester. However, after that first year, I had to drop out again for more surgery on my hips. As a result, my college career went from the age of 20 or 19, through to 25, because I was in and out of the hospital during that time. When I finally graduated I had several plays under my belt and I had performed once in New York. I auditioned for another show in New York and got that.

The first show was a musical piece called Viet Rock, which toured to three different regional theatres, and then off-Broadway at The Chekhov Studios named after Michael Chekhov, the acting teacher. Viet Rock was very much an ensemble piece with each cast member playing multiple parts. In act one I was a recruit and draftee to show how the Vietnam War did not always discern disability as a factor for the draft. In act two I was head of the Viet Cong (played entirely by the women in the cast), a role I created as assistant director of the piece. Then I did another show in New York called the *Soda Jerk*, which I auditioned for just before I graduated. I was the 'ghost' of a superhero sidekick from an old TV show who appeared as an advisor in a moment of crisis.

And then the decision was, do I go to New York, or do I go to Los Angeles? It was literally a coin toss. We had visited a friend of mine in San Diego, which is about a two-hour drive south of Los Angeles. We liked the weather so much, and, of course, at the time the girls, so we ended up choosing Los Angeles. I got there at the end of 1989, and that was the era of literally pounding the pavement, going door to door, knocking on agents' doors and trying to get myself recognised. There was no internet. There was no way to circulate my material, which meant that I literally had to walk the pavement and see who might be interested in me. I walked into many different agencies.

I joined a now defunct agency in San Diego, but they never really did anything for me. Then I heard of the Coralie Jr. agency. The agency once repped Cuba Gooding Jr, who thanked the agency in his Oscar speech. The agency also provided little people with work. I got with that agency and they got me a job as a costume character. It was a non-union job for about a month and paid $300 a day. It was a big deal back in 1990. Then I was doing stand-in work and learning a lot in the course of being on set and observing. I was never one to go away and come back later. I just stayed and watched to try to learn as much as I could, and I probably learnt more in a year just being on set than I did in four years of being in film school. Instead of just learning about theory I was learning the whole technical side and day to day of how things are done.

Getting Roles

I was in a show called Pros and Cons with James Earl Jones and Richard Crenna. *Pros and Cons* (1991–1992) was an American crime drama series about Gabriel Bird (James Earl Jones), a police officer who had been wrongly sentenced to life imprisonment for the murder of a fellow officer. I played a giant strawberry in a big bowl of Cornflakes for a Cornflakes commercial. It was this play within a play, which was my first experience with a television show with an enormous budget. They built this enormous cereal bowl and put all these gigantic Cornflakes in, and then put me in as a talking strawberry. It was absurd, and it was fun, but I only got the role because I was small and I could fit into the costume.

At this time, Danny was getting roles that required the use of someone with dwarfism to fill a costume, as opposed to being given a role based on his acting abilities. I then landed a role as a costumed character on an episode of *Murder, She Wrote*. Murder, She Wrote was an American crime drama television series that ran from 1984 to 1996. The show starred Angela Lansbury as Jessica Fletcher, a retired teacher and amateur detective. In Murder on Madison Avenue (Season 8, episode 22), I played the uncredited 'Gunslinger robot', who drew a gun on Jessica Fletcher. I was a costumed character that did not have any lines. Before computer-generated imagery (CGI), due to their stature, little people were often cast as costume characters. Some of the most notable costume characters fulfiled by little people include E.T. (*E.T. the Extra-Terrestrial*), Ewoks (*Star Wars*) and the Goblins of Gringotts Wizarding Bank (*Harry Potter*) to name but a few. In most cases, the role does not involve much dialogue, reducing the person with dwarfism to someone who fulfils the movement of a prop.

If you are an extra or a costumed character, there is an unwritten rule that you never cross the line into the other world of all the A-listers and the series regulars, but I was never one to pay attention to that. I would just interact like a normal person and 1 day I got to talking to Angela Lansbury and she liked my humour. Dame Angela Lansbury (1925–2022) was an award-winning film, television and stage actress, with a career that spanned over 80 years. To be recognised by Angela Lansbury is certainly a career boost. Angela Lansbury was the first person who saw me as an actor and gave me the opportunity to come in and do something real. She invited me back to do two more episodes as a speaking character. The first time I played a Greek landlord, Giorgi Pappavasilopoulos in The Sound of Murder (Season 9, Episode 10). Then I came back and played Mr Townsend in A Virtual Murder (Season 10, episode 5). I found it remarkable for someone like Angela Lansbury to want to hire somebody like me (a little person) in the early 1990s. She was, I think, the first person that I ran into who did not see me as this other thing. While Angela Lansbury was open minded regarding what an actor with dwarfism could be, others still regarded people with dwarfism as figures of fun who could not possibly work in everyday occupations.

Avoiding Stereotypes

Throughout the 1990s there were a lot of shows based on particular stereotypes of little people, but there was also slight deviation. I was getting calls for a lot of roles, usually for a character that was volatile or violent. A funny thing about the 1990s was that a lot of these episodes that focused on little people had funny names in their titles. For example, it could be 'Small Packages' or 'A Little Murder'. They make a point to say something about size. In relation to little people, there is often an emphasis placed on their stature. This behaviour reflects notions of the freak show, where a little person's stature was the sole purpose of their performance. Providing titles to shows that focus on stature when a little person is featured, gives the message that height is in itself a form of amusement that is enough to entice viewers.

Most people with dwarfism work in everyday occupations, including within medicine, such as William Shakespeare (Physician), Judith Badner (Geneticist and Psychiatrist) and Michael Ain (Paediatric Orthopaedic Surgeon), to name but a few. However, general society still considers people with dwarfism to be figures of entertainment and cannot envisage them as being capable of working in professions, such as medicine.

I remember asking my agent to pitch me for a doctor role in ER. ER was an American medical drama television series that ran from 1994 to 2009. It remains NBC's third longest running drama (Keveney, 2005) and is available on some streaming services. The show's popularity could have shown the general public how a career in medicine is available to little people, challenging the belief that we are reliant on work in the entertainment industry. The feedback I got back was, 'Oh, he, he! Someone like him could never be a doctor'. At the time I knew who Michael Ain was, and I said to the ER people, 'I know somebody who's studying to be a doctor, who is becoming an orthopaedic surgeon and who is going to be working at Johns Hopkins Hospital and he has achondroplasia'. Some doctors are little people in the world, but once they say no, they do not want to hear the rest of your argument.

There was that dichotomy of, there are so many things I could do, but, there were still some areas that were off-limits. I remember as a young kid, my neighbour said to me, 'Do you know what are you gonna do with your life?' I said, 'Well, I don't know. I think I might do this, or whatever', I said. And he goes 'Well, you could never be a truck driver'. He was one of those kinds of kids like, 'I'm gonna be a trucker', and I said, 'Well, not that I want to be a truck driver, but I'm sure that if I did want to be a truck driver I would do it'. He said, 'Well you couldn't get your hands around the wheel'. He was dead set against the idea of me being a truck driver. Fast forward in my career years and I played truck driver. That was me getting the last laugh after all these years. You would not have seen that you would not have seen that 20 years ago you just would not have and there are a lot of things you would not see then.

A lot of times the roles would come to me that had this pathos around shame, and that I do not like who I am because of my size. There was this one show in particular. It was one of these late-night cable channels, what they called 'jiggle shows'. A jiggle show refers to programs that rely heavily on the sexuality of young women to entice viewers (Jezierski, 2011). It was called *Silk Stalkings: Passion and the Palm Beach Detectives* (Series 8, Episode 3). *Silk Stalkings* was an American crime drama television series that ran from 1991 to1999. It was a provocative programme on cable, but there was no nudity, just all the suggestions of nudity. It was a popular cable show and I was invited to play a character called Sherman Bisco who was a romance novelist and murderer.

The way the script ended was that the reason I was a murderer was because I was ashamed or humiliated because of my size. I said that it was not realistic.

People like me (little people) are not ashamed to be small. We accept who we are. Anything that comes at us is external, it is not internal. It all comes from society's perceptions and has nothing to do with how we feel about ourselves subjectively. It is about our objectification from the outside, how we are perceived and what society labels us as. I said, 'Look, I don't want to do this the way it's written'. This was the time when I could make some changes and occasionally the writers and producers would listen. I gave them a whole sort of premise about who my character was. He was a cuckold husband, who was a ghostwriter for his wife, who became a famous author, but she was just living the good life of a rich woman who got a lot of money from her husband's work. I was cuckolded and playing like the butler to her, and she was humiliating me that way, but it had no mention of my size ever throughout this entire episode. That is the way to go. It is not about that shame. It is about the way the wife was treating him and that is why he becomes this killer. It was one of those episodes where I could make a difference. I could talk to the producers and the writers, and make changes that worked for me, but that has not always been the case.

I was asked to do the Television series, *Honey. I Shrunk the Kids*, which first aired in 1997 and ran for three consecutive seasons. The television series was based on the 1989 comedy film of the same name. The show was about a scientist father who accidentally shrinks his teenage children and two other neighbourhood teens to the size of insects. In season 2, episode 10, *Honey, I've Joined the Big Top*, there was a character who was in a circus. I thought, Okay, I can get on board with the circus. I knew little people were circus performers at the time. I know they existed. I guess it is a stereotypical role, but if there is some substance to it, I can work with that and the characters throughout this episode.

It is a children's comedy television series and my role involved my character playing 'kissy face' with the 14-year-old daughter of the family. He is constantly trying to kiss her. I thought that was really creepy because at the time I was a man in my 30s. I said, 'There's no way this would ever happen. I would never do that without being arrested'. I asked for it to be removed from the storyline, but they refused and found somebody else for the role. People with dwarfism are often infantilised and when it comes to sexuality, they are often deemed asexual or hypersexual (Pritchard, 2021). In this case, the character with dwarfism, that Danny was asked to play, would be both hypersexual and asexual. He would be hypersexual in the way he chases a young girl for kisses, but deemed asexual so as not to take this inappropriate act as threatening. The fact that people with dwarfism are often infantilised would construct the character as childlike, and thus there would be less emphasis that a man was sexually harassing a young girl.

Characters with dwarfism are often expected to engage in practices that would be off-limits to other characters. Engaging with practices that would not be expected from other adult men implies that some producers do not deem people with dwarfism to be fully human. Rather, they are constructed as a nuisance, unable to control their behaviour, which challenges societal norms. There is this idea that little people are like animals and it makes me cringe. I can recall at least three times when I have been asked to bite somebody. I auditioned for a role in the American family drama *Picket Fences* (1992–1996). The audition required my character to bite the lead actress's backside. My character bites her on the backside and then he asks her on the date, and then she says, yes. I said, 'that it would never happen. I'd be arrested. I'd be slapped'. I told them that it was creepy and painted this picture of little people as being animalistic. It paints little people, especially men as sexual deviants. Instead of having a sensuality, little people men are aligned with an overt sexual predilection or fetish. It just did not sit right with me. I asked the casting director at the time if we could change it as it was not something that I was comfortable doing. Their response was 'No, that's how it's written. That's how it's going to be'. I knew that the writer of this was notorious for sticking to his script as written. Again, somebody else did it that way and I was mortified for them. I was also angry that this type of behaviour and representation of little people was being perpetuated.

My rebellion in this regard comes from what gets perpetuated about little people, especially men who are little people. The women with dwarfism, I know in this industry, get even fewer roles. But at that time, Debbie Lee Carrington (1959–2018) was the main go to woman with dwarfism. I think a lot of times they wanted to do what they could to sexualise her. Her first breakout was *Total Recall* (1990) in which she plays a prostitute and the novelty of that is almost like it is titillating and laughable at the same time. I think that the way that they see little people with regards to sex, it is titillating and laughable simultaneously. Dwarfism and sexuality seem to have an incongruous relationship. People with dwarfism are already constructed as figures of fun, but the idea that they can participate in sexual activities is unexpected and further becomes a point of humour.

I was then offered a part in the Christmas movie *Jingle All the Way* (1996). There was a fight sequence in the film where we were coming up with things to do, and the director said, 'You know I want you to run up and in this scene and bite Arnold (Schwarzenegger) on the butt'. That hit me in the gut, and I said, 'I don't want to do that'. This was my first major role in a big-budget film, and I thought I needed to be able to tell him that it was not what I wanted to do. I do not want to have that depiction go out there. I was grateful enough that the director understood and that I wanted another option to not have to do that because I found it humiliating. I found it degrading to little people. It was up to me to come up with an alternative. I asked for a stun gun and pitched that idea instead, to zap him (Arnold Schwarzenegger) instead of biting him like an animal.

I was offered a role straight out for a sitcom called *Hope and Faith* (2003–2006). However, the script stated that I was to bite the lead actor on the leg in a fight sequence. Again, I refused. I thought I do not want to get to New York and have the director say, 'Well, it was in the script, we're going to do it that way'. As a result, I told my agent at the time, to put in the contract, that there would be no biting of any kind during this filming. I wanted to make sure that it did not get thrown back in my face. They might agree to it now, but then they might change their mind and want me to do it.

I have been threatened to be sent home or fired if I did not consent to certain depictions, one of which was a character I was portraying who was asked to be in a child's seat in the car. I said, 'I'm not going to do that'. Even though I was playing this otherworldly creature, I did not want to be in a child's seat. I did not want to have that depiction because ultimately people relate that to someone who is perceived as an adult but small, so they should fit in a child's seat. It was meant for comedy, not for safety. I refused to do that. I told the producers that it was not a portrayal I wanted to do. It became an agreement I made with them before taking the role. It was just a verbal agreement I had with them. However, on the pilot test the prop guy came in to give me a choice of child seating for the scene. I said, 'No, that's been cut'. He leaves, and then the producer comes in and says, 'Oh, yeah, that we're still doing that'. I said, 'No cause as we agreed, I wouldn't be doing that'. Later he returns and says, 'The network says if you don't do it, they are going to send you home'. This was the test, to remind me that I have the job, but it still could go away. So I just took off my apron from the makeup chair, got up and I said, 'Well, send me home'. And then he said, 'Well, hold on'. Then he went away, and then later came back, and said, 'It's fine you don't have to do the child seat'. It was a threat that you are going to lose your job if you do not do what we say. It implied that I was a problem, even though the agreement was made prior to me taking the role. These are experiences that have come my way, and I have had to address them on set in that particular moment.

Seinfeld

Seinfeld is an American sitcom that ran from 1989 to 1998. The show centres on the main character, comedian Jerry Seinfeld, his friends and neighbours, in New York. Danny played Mickey Abbot, who was born to average sized parents and objected to being referred to as a 'midget'. This representation of a character with dwarfism helps to challenge two problematic beliefs associated with dwarfism in society. Eighty percent of people with dwarfism are born to average sized parents; however, due to depictions of dwarfism as a separate race (see, *Snow White and the Seven Dwarfs*, *Charlie and the Chocolate Factory* and *The Wizard of Oz*), people often assume that our families are also little people. Having the opportunity to challenge the word midget in the show is a good way of educating millions of viewers that people with dwarfism do not find this term acceptable.

In regards to my role as Mickey Abbott in Seinfeld, I think it was the first time that there was a character who was part of a collective, a friend of the group. Except for the first episode there were never any other moments or reason to address Mickey's height. I think to normalise his presence in the show was a big step in the 1990s. He is sort of likeable and not likeable in many respects. All Seinfeld characters in general are pretty unlikable people. They have those idiosyncrasies that make them disagreeable in so many ways. They are always sort of complaining about one thing or another. They are uncomfortable in society and that dislike sometimes would set him off, and he would get angry and volatile. Mickey was sort of falling into the trap because he was Kramer's friend.

Every time I got a script I would be nervous paging through it, thinking that I am going to find something that is objectionable. For the first 20 years of my career, I go to the script and look for something that is objectionable, because a lot of times I would find it and that was the thing about Seinfeld, I never found it.

I was sensitive to a lot of these things because of what I have experienced in my life and what I experienced in other shows, how they would portray little people. It never was like that. So I think they were advanced in that regard to just create this character and let him be.

I think that was the most innovative thing about my character. They created this character, and yes, he is a little person, and yes, we utilise that aspect in the first episode, but it was never a big storyline, but rather used in more subtle ways. For example, Kramer asked me, stand in for the little kid when he goes to find the boy that is missing, and I fall asleep waiting for him to come back pretending to be the boy asleep, and then the mother comes home and finds me in the bed asleep, and loses her mind. You know little little things like that, but I never found any of that to be offencive or objectionable to me as a man, you know, or as a person with dwarfism. These were just sort of real possibilities that could have been mirrored in real life, not something forced or made up, or stereotypical. Seinfeld gave me a fully fleshed out character and started to show that I could play other roles.

Paying the Price

I think there are very few actors that have to deal with being stereotyped in the way little people are, who get put in these positions where their power is taken away. Little people in the entertainment industry are often humiliated or laughed at. I know, there are plenty of little people, actors that have done things that I would never do. However, in my opinion, we should never put the person not in power in that position that they should be ashamed. They are maybe even much smaller than me, which means that they have a whole different outlook. I think certain heights of dwarfism have differing responses. For example, I remember Verne Troyer telling the story of someone picking him up and carrying him across the street because he was standing at a corner.[1] He did not even want to cross the street. I think his life perspective, being more vulnerable, affected his outlook and his survival instincts. Thus, while I would not agree to these roles, there are little people who will agree to do them. I just try not to judge their life. I am more prone to judging the producers and the writers of such a role.

I remember, one character was offered to me on a show. For the role, I would walk around with a tray of hors d'oeuvres on my head. There was not really much else to the role, but the character was guaranteed to come back in several episodes. I could just see that it was going to be an ongoing site gag where the character is humiliated a lot. It is not something I wanted to be associated with at all. But I knew a guy who was much smaller than me, who did the role and while I did not like that he did it, I could not necessarily call him out. I could call out the writers, cause I think they are always gonna find somebody who will do these roles, because for little people, too, you want to work. You want to make enough

---

[1] Verne Troyer (1969–2018) was an actor with dwarfism, most notable for playing mini-Me in the Austin Powers Trilogy (1997–2002).

money to get insurance. This is your sole income as a performer, as an actor. You do not want to have to leave it.

I have seen enough tragedy. In this industry there has been a number of suicides of little people. One that stands out in my mind is David Steinberg, who was in the 1988 fantasy film *Willow*. David also starred in numerous television shows, such as the children's horror television series, *Are You Afraid of the Dark?* (1990–1996). He struggled after a while because he had two things going on. One, he was a little person and two he had lost a lot of family, including his partner. He was also gay and, being a little person, was not a great combination either in terms of being accepted by society.

David had been invited to do a soap opera called *Passions* (1999–2007). He was, I think, overwhelmed by the amount of lines and work his role involved. Unfortunately, he did not have the confidence to talk to the producers and tell them that he needed more time, or any adaptations. He had no real support system at the time. So, day 1 he just decided not to show up for work. He missed out on all that work. It was about 26 episodes. I had done the role to replace him, but I did not know who they replaced at the time. I just knew that they were replacing somebody, and then I found out later that it was him.

I saw him at an audition, and I talked to him for a bit, and I could see he was upset. He was sad. He told me how much he was struggling financially. He was trying to get a job as a hotel concierge, and you know he was also struggling physically because he also had Spondyloepiphyseal Dysplasia Congenita (SEDc).[2] His life was tougher as he got older and eventually it just became too much for him, especially without a support team in place. He took his own life shortly after that audition where I saw him.

That was a tragedy, and you can not say you blame this business because this business is tough all around, but at the same time it is tougher for somebody like him who does not have the opportunity to go get another job, such as a delivery person for United Parcel Service (UPS). There is a lot more struggles for little people to maintain other employment.

In this industry, people often do other work. It is not necessarily skilled labour, although they require skill sets. They want to at the very least try to keep a roof over their head. David had gone to college and actually spent a semester at my school. I met him there when I was in college and he offered me something he was also doing at the time. There is the big annual Radio City Christmas show where they use a lot of little people called Radio City Rockettes. I remember David was going off to do Willow, and he stopped me and he said, 'Do you want to do a role with Radio City?' I was like a big fish in a small pond, and I said 'I was not gonna be an Elf, I did not want to do that. I know it's $700. Blah! Blah! Blah! But I'm gonna go be a movie star somewhere'. So I turned it down, which, for me at the time, was the right choice. Gary Arnold, another little person, recalls that they were hired as Elves and unlike the other Rockettes, who were dancers, were hired for their skills, the little people were not (Arnold, 2012). It was back in the 1980s

---

[2] A form of dwarfism with numerous secondary conditions.

and you got $700 a week, which was a huge amount back then. It was something that you could certainly survive on. However, the Radio City work is not doable all year long and thus is a precarious occupation.

David went from that from doing films to doing other things, including television to just not working, to just not being called. I know that this business can turn around in a second. Over my career I have been able to build other areas of my skill set with regard to consulting with studios on disability and employment. I get to do that as well as this. At the same time, my desire is always to get back to film and television.

The Woodburn Ratio

Danny's attitude as an actor who refuses roles that perpetuate problematic stereotypes of dwarfism, as well his insights into how the industry is more limiting in terms of opportunities for disabled actors, has made him activist.

In recent years Danny has been a strong critic of the practice of 'cripping up'. Cripping up refers to a non-disabled actor playing a character with a disability. There are two main criticisms of cripping up. Firstly, from an economic perspective, the practice denies actors with a disability a role that would otherwise provide financial support. This is even more problematic when cripping up is argued to be a practice where an actor is cast to play a character from a less dominant social position (Sandahl, 2008). Secondly, cripping up impacts how people with disabilities are represented.

In relation to cripping up, I have what I call the 'Woodburn ratio'. I came up with this idea after a conversation between me and Bryan Cranston. Bryan had starred in The Upside, a comedy drama film where he plays Philip Lacasse, who is quadriplegic. There was a lot of backlash from the disability community about that. After criticisms towards Bryan's role in the film, the actor responded to critics by claiming that it had been a business decision (Dry, 2019). It is his name, Bryan Cranston in The Upside, making him the marquee for the film. A marquee refers to an actor who can bring in large audiences. Due to Bryan Cranston's success in numerous films and television shows, including Breaking Bad (2008–2013), any show featuring him is likely to pull in a large audience.

I had brought it up to him (Bryan), and he said, 'Well, the press team sort of handled it. It is sort of behind us now'. And I said, 'Well, it's not behind you, because it still exists in the disability community, and there's still a lot of hurt in the community, and I wonder if you would talk to me about it'. He agreed, and (I) talked to him about why it is difficult for the disability community to accept disabled characters being played by non-disabled actors.

I agree that on one hand, actors should be allowed to play whomever they want to play. But the opposing argument to that is a lot of disabled actors are not getting the opportunity to play whatever they want to play. It is not because they are not talented. It is not because they are not capable. It is because they are not given the opportunity to grow, to progress, to become an A list, or to become, as he says, he is a marquee. People with disabilities are less likely to get access to education and in this arena they are less likely to be employed, less likely to get representation. They are less likely to continue to work in their craft like I talked to him about. You have really got to make your mark and be recognised.

The stage is not fully accessible to everybody. For example, The Second City in Hollywood, was an old building with no elevator, just a huge flight of stairs that led to the rehearsal space and the performance space.[3] It means that if you are a wheelchair user you are not getting up there. If you have a mobility disability that makes stairs difficult to navigate, then you are not getting up there. Once you are in there you then have to get up and down off the stage – up and down, off the stage.

When Ali Stroker was in *Oklahoma!* and won a Tony Award, two things happened.[4] One, when she did Oklahoma, they built the stage so that she could get on and off very easily. They also built a dressing room for her that she could get in and out of that was accessible with an accessible bathroom. These are not in all theatres. I explained this to Bryan Cranston – how disabled people are not going to get those opportunities, and we are not going to be searched for.

Bryan gets to go to work. He gets to be a disabled character, but at the end of the day he is going to be able to walk up on stage. He is Bryan Cranston, and he does not have a disability. When somebody with a disability portrays a character with a disability, and they win an award, there is a visceral feeling. For example, when Marlee Matlin won her Academy Award, they (film critic Rex Reed) said she should not have won because she is Deaf. In 1986, film critic Rex Reed claimed that Marlee had won the award out of pity and questioned how a Deaf actor playing a Deaf person was actually acting (Clarke, 2021). Reed's comment implies that an actor who plays the role of a disabled character is only playing the disability, which neglects all other attributes of that character, as well as being able to portray various emotions. It was as if her deafness was the only quality that she had. The way that actors with disabilities are identified is just by disability. Little people are identified just by their dwarfism. It is always "you can not", or "how can you?" Reed's attitude reflects the dominant attitude towards disability within the entertainment industry. The Academy Awards has a history of rewarding non-disabled actors for playing characters with disabilities (Lindner, 2015). For example, Dustin Hoffman, Tom Hanks and Eddie Redmayne have all won Oscars for their portrayal of a character with a disability. While over 20 non-disabled actors have won Oscars for playing disabled characters, only two actors with disabilities have won Oscars (Dry, 2019).[5]

After our conversation, Bryan said, 'Well, how can I change it?' I said, 'Well, in the future, if you get an opportunity like this where you are going to take this role away from a person with a disability you have to give three back'. If you are going to give the role of a character with disability to a non-disabled person, you have to give three speaking roles in your film or television show to disabled performers. That is my Woodburn ratio. The aim is to elevate them and move actors with disabilities into the A-list sphere, this marquee sphere, this high-echelon paid performer. There are very few of us and I think at the end of the day someone with Marley Matlins' career is still

---

[3]Closed in 2022, The Second City specialised in comedy theatre.
[4]First wheelchair users to win a Tony Award.
[5]Three since Troy Kurtsur won an Oscar for the 2021 film CODA.

probably paid less than somebody with an equivalent career, but who is not Deaf. That is my guess. I am making an assumption there, of course.

Instead of producers asking 'How can you do this?' Or 'How can you play this role?' They should be asking 'How can we get you to do this role?' 'How can we make this role more accessible?' That way it becomes a joint effort on everybody's part. I always cite the Green M&M's scenario, where some upper echelon performers, to make sure that their contracts are followed to the T, throw in some extraneous thing in their contract. For example, they might write in their contract that there must be a bowl of green M&M's in their dressing room every day when they show up. However, this request is more likely to be ensured than providing an accessible bathroom for a disabled actor. Every makeup trailer and wardrobe trailer that I have ever been in has three to five steps going up inside from outside. I have pulled myself up and down those steps for three decades now, but only when I can.

I remember when I was doing Seinfeld. There were several dressing rooms outside that were for all the main characters, and rightfully so they are in and out much more frequently than all us guest actors. But my dressing room was outside across this one driveway, and then up three flights of stairs to the top of this old building, where they had a row of guest dressing rooms. I said to the producers, 'If I go out there between the scenes, go all the way up there to change my wardrobe and then come back, you're gonna be waiting a long time to get me back on stage'. So I said, 'Just build a screen here on the soundstage. I'll go in the corner. I'll change my clothes. That's fine. I don't care'. I have worked in the theatre where I have stripped down, and got dressed again in front of whomever was there, so I did not care about that. What I wanted to avoid was having to run up and down those stairs. It is like half a day's work, to do all that every time between scenes. That was an accommodation that I asked for and it was not a big deal. Some accommodations can be met and done, which are not a big deal.

After 100-plus years of filmmaking and 33 years of the Americans with Disabilities Act 1990, it is time to make sure that these reasonable accommodations are there for disabled performers and not an afterthought. They should be part of the production. Even if they do not think that they are going to hire an actor with a disability it should be part of the discussion, anyway, part of production meetings or studio objectives. If you do not make it part of the discussion, then you say that when an actor with a disability wants an opportunity, they will say, 'Oh, well, we can't use them, because this is up inside a house. It's an old house. We have no way to get them up'. It is about preparing ahead of time for the possibility that you have a disabled performer on a show. I think that is integral to the advancement of our society as a whole because it will make other businesses think the same thing, you know. It is always about adapting and making accommodations. It is about the possibilities. Were there? What is that? You know?

Conclusion

Danny has had and continues to have a successful career in the entertainment industry. However, his path to success has not been easy, due to the problematic beliefs many producers have about dwarfism, and thus how they think dwarfism should be represented in their films or television shows. In numerous cases, producers have a very problematic view of dwarfism which can influence problematic perceptions about dwarfism in society. While Danny does not believe that actors with dwarfism pursuing these roles should be blamed for perpetuating stereotypes, we need to recognise that producers will continue to hold these beliefs unless they are challenged.

This chapter has also shown how some people in the entertainment industry are open to providing more positive representations of dwarfism.

Danny's experiences have provided a detailed insight into the numerous attitudinal and physical barriers that disabled people encounter within the entertainment industry. In particular, the physical barriers actors with disabilities encounter, instead of being removed, producers have instead opted for cripping up. To avoid cripping up, we need to go back to basics and consider the access needs of actors with disabilities. If studios can create elaborate fantasy worlds, then it should not be too hard to include a few accommodations for actors with disabilities.

References

Adelson, B. (2005). *The lives of dwarfs: Their journey from public curiosity toward social liberation*. Rutgers University Press.

Arnold, G. (2012). Radio city style evolution. *LPA Blogspot* [online]. https://dwarfism-lpa.blogspot.com/2012/12/radio-city-style-evolution.html. Accessed on January 12, 2024.

Clarke, C. (2021). 'Deaf is not a costume': Marlee Matlin on surviving abuse and casting authentically. *The Guardian* [online]. https://www.theguardian.com/film/2021/aug/06/deaf-is-not-a-costume-marlee-matlin-on-surviving-abuse-and-casting-authentically. Accessed on December 05, 2023.

Dry, J. (2019). Bryan Cranston signed on to 'the upside' knowing his casting was problematic — Here's why. *Indie Wire* [online]. https://www.indiewire.com/features/general/bryan-cranston-interview-the-upside-disabled-actors-opportunities-1202033892/. Accessed on December 07, 2023.

Jezierski, A. (2011). *Television everywhere: How Hollywood can take back the internet and turn digital dimes into dollars*. Iuniverse Inc.

Keveney, D. (2005). After 11 years, Dr. Carter takes leave from 'ER'. *Wayback Machine* [online]. https://web.archive.org/web/20090709102637/http://www.erheadquarters.com/news/11/after11years_033105.htm. Accessed on January 11, 2024.

Lindner, K. (2015). Why are we so surprised at the Oscars' lack of diversity? *The Conversation* [online]. https://theconversation.com/why-are-we-so-surprised-at-the-oscars-lack-of-diversity-36029. Accessed on December 07, 2023.

Pritchard, E. (2021). The metanarrative of dwarfism. In D. Bolt (Ed.), *The metanarrative of disability* (pp. 123–137). Routledge.

Raynor, O., & Hayward, K. (2009). Breaking into the business: Experiences of actors with disabilities in the entertainment industry. *Journal of Research in Special Educational Needs*, 9(1), 39–47.

Sandahl, C. (2008). Why disability identity matters: From dramaturgy to casting in John Belluso's Pyretown. *Text and Performance Quarterly*, 28(1), 225–241.

Chapter 7

Get the Balance Right: The Change in How People With Dwarfism Are Depicted From Limited, Damaging and Negative to Realistic, Creative and Positive

Simon Minty (Producer of Abnormally Funny People and Board Member of the National Theatre)

UK

> Once you've accepted your flaws, no one can use them against you. (Tyrion Lannister, Game of Thrones, Season 2, Episode 1: The North Remembers)

I feel 'wince' is an underutilised word. As a child of the 1970s and 1980s, however, I found I used it a lot. Back then, whenever someone who had dwarfism came on my television screen, I would wince. Reflecting on why, I think there were two reasons. One, the lesser of the two, was because of something known as the mirror image effect. I have dwarfism. I would see someone short and realise that is how I look to others. It is an unavoidable reminder that the self-image I had in my head was not the same as how I look in reality. I was growing up, and my identity was being formed, informed by different images. My self-image did not include how I walked or my body shape with its bumps and curves in non-typical places. It did not show the difference between me and someone average sized. I would see someone else with dwarfism, and I did not recognise myself or I did not want to. Yet, seeing someone else with the rare condition I had, I could not dismiss it.

The bigger, more impactful wince was from their depiction. If I struggled to recognise their body shape, I absolutely did not recognise their behaviour. There was not a character or individual I can recall whose height went unmentioned or was unremarkable. Height difference was rarely treated with respect or seriousness. More likely, there would be a joke about their height in a comedy sketch by some like Benny Hill or they would be dressed as a fantasy or mythical creature such as The Munchkins in *The Wizard of Oz* or an Ewok in *Star Wars*. The dwarfism was the point of amusement, not underlying talent or person. Rarely was it ever

---

Dwarfism Arts and Advocacy, 89–100
Copyright © 2024 Simon Minty
Published under exclusive licence by Emerald Publishing Limited
doi:10.1108/978-1-83753-922-220241016

'normal'. Seeing myself like this, on screen or stage, during my critical childhood years was hard. I am sure it had a deep impact, some of which I have explored later as an adult. This was a conflict between my own self-image and self-worth compared to what was shown. It did not make sense to me. It has driven me to try and make a change.

Today, I do not see as many jokes about dwarfism on television or film. It is not gone, but it is less so. There is still a fair bit of fantasy or creature work for people with dwarfism, but today, I do not wince so much. My reaction is complex. A mixture of feeling punch-drunk, stoical and if really bad and offensive, raging with fury.

> A wise man once said that the true history of the world is the history of great conversations in elegant rooms. (Tyrion Lannister, Game of Thrones, Season 6, Episode 3: Oathbreaker)

My name is Simon Minty. I am a self-employed consultant and trainer, running my own small and successful consultancy business. I deliver training on disability in the workplace, training managers and disabled colleagues. In addition, I am on two boards, as a Non-executive Director of Motability Operations plc, a UK car leasing company for disabled people, and on the Board of Directors at the National Theatre in London. I co-host a monthly podcast called *The Way We Roll* which explores all things related to disability. In 2005, I co-created a team of comedians called *Abnormally Funny People*. Abnormally Funny People is a loose collective of professional comedians, all of whom have a disability of some sort.

I am a cast member of the television show *Gogglebox* (2013-present) with my sister Jane. Every Friday night, for 30 weeks a year, I pop up on television on Channel 4 [British free-to-air public broadcast television channel], one of the main television stations in the United Kingdom. It is a hugely popular show and, according to MostlyMedia, at its peak during the pandemic; *Gogglebox* drew in an audience of between 5 and 6 million. Viewership now hovers consistently around the 4 million mark, and since 2014, it has featured religiously in Channel 4's top five programmes (Mostly Media, 2023). I sit on a sofa, with my average-height sister Jane, and we make comments about television shows we are watching together. The viewer essentially watches us watching television.

I cannot list every key person and every key moment that has led to the current approach to how dwarfism and disability are depicted on screen. I cannot list every project I have been part of. It is more than a chapter, and I am grateful other writers are creating brilliant chapters alongside this one. Instead, I will explore what I think are some of the key moments and the projects I have been involved in. The credit goes to everyone.

> That's what I do: I drink and I know things. (Tyrion Lannister, Game of Thrones, Season 6, Episode 3: Oathbreaker)

Most people know the actor Peter Dinklage, via his epic role being Tyrion Lannister in the hugely popular *Game of Thrones* series (2011–2019). Not everyone knows how he got there, his approach to acting as someone with dwarfism. I first came across him in the satirical black comedy film Living in Oblivion (1995). A close friend from my school days alerted me to this film, explaining 'There is a character in it saying what you say' about representation. *Living in Oblivion* is a film about making a film. Dinklage's character, Tito, plays a 'dwarf representing anxiety' in a dream sequence. In this scene, we see Dinklage holding aloft an apple while walking around the lead character. He is dressed in sky blue tails and a sky blue top hat. After a few takes, clearly unhappy, Tito challenges the director of the fake film (played by Steve Buscemi) with the astute question, 'Why does my character have to be a dwarf? Have you ever had a dream with a dwarf in it? Do you know anyone who has had a dream with a dwarf in it? I don't even dream with dwarfs in it' (Living in Oblivion, 1995). He implies the only reason he is there is to make it 'weird' and the only time dwarfs appear in dreams is in 'stupid movies like this'. I watched this and marvelled. It was true, a character was saying what I was thinking. In case you are wondering, I do dream about other dwarfs, but that is because they are my friends and real people.

Dinklage next appeared on my radar in the comedy/drama film, The Station Agent (2003). I understand this role was written for him. He plays Finbar, a recluse, someone who loves trains but avoids the public as the treatment of him has not been favourable. His circumstances change and he moves house. In his new place, he is exposed to new people and dragged into the real world he has been avoiding. Dinklage plays the role with understatement; he is quiet, detached and does not want to be around people. I am an extrovert I am permanently on display and often attract attention, so I love this character as I yearn to be it sometimes. The pivotal scene for me is in a bar where already tired, Finbar drinks, smokes and ruminates. People stare at him with a mix of curiosity, mocking and sympathy. He then explodes, jumping up on a bar stool, arms aloft, looking at everyone and shouts, 'Here I am! Look. Take a look' (The Station Agent, 2003). He stumbles down from the stool, and one of the people previously staring at him comes to support him, preventing him from falling over. It is an unsettling scene. It is one that I have experienced a few times in my life, without the drinking and smoking, where I have been driven to the point of challenging the staring people to ask, 'This is it, what else do you want from me?' (The Station Agent, 2003).

To continue the Dinklage homage, he plays the career-defining Tyrion Lannister in *Game of Thrones*. His character is hugely complex, a drinker, a sexual being, an intellectual, an advisor, someone who reads and someone who is ignored. His height is both critical and incidental. I could pull out a dozen moments that had an impact on me and I hope affected how other people view those of us with dwarfism. But I will go with one when he is on trial for a murder he did not commit. While defending himself, he has a charged conversation with his father Tywin, who is also the unfavourably biased judge. After berating and alienating the crowd who have gathered to watch, he continues.

> *Tyrion Lannister:* I wish... to confess. I saved you. I saved this city and all your worthless lives. I should have let Stannis kill you all. I am guilty. Guilty. Is that what you want to hear?
>
> *Tywin Lannister:* You admit you poisoned the king?

> *Tyrion Lannister:* No, of that I am innocent. I am guilty of a far more monstrous crime. I am guilty of being a dwarf.
>
> *Tywin Lannister:* You are not on trial for being a dwarf.
>
> *Tyrion Lannister:* Oh, yes, I am. I've been on trial for that my entire life. (The Laws of Gods and Men, 2014)

Hearing this line was like a whack around the head, a shock to the heart and a grabbing of my soul. I did not know whether to laugh or cry. I wanted to hug Tyrion and salute the scriptwriter. It was something I had never articulated, and yet the words made absolute sense. Tyrion is saying this trial is about him being different. When you are a person with dwarfism, everyone notices you are different and looks at you. Whatever you do, wherever you go people stare, are curious, overly friendly or sometimes rude. Back in reality, when I go to the supermarket, I get attention and if I choose, direct eye contact with 20 people, 10 smiles, multiple unnatural non-responses. At times, my life has felt like I am on one long trial. More accurately, I often feel like I am an Ambassador as if I represent all people with dwarfism. There are so few of us, that how I behave will reflect on all of us. That is why I feel I am permanently on trial.

In 2021, Dinklage got to be the lead in *Cyrano*, a major feature film. He played Cyrano in the film adaptation of the play, Cyrano de Bergerac. In an ingenious and apt twist, Dinklage's Cyrano never 'gets the girl' supposedly because of his height, not because of the size of his nose as in the original Cyrano. Cyrano has the words, the wit and the wisdom to woo her but sacrifices his desires to help another man. I have played this role in real life. While the film did not change the world, someone with dwarfism being backed as the male romantic lead in a film is significant. It demonstrates that we are not asexual but also showcases some of the prejudices people hold against people with dwarfism when it comes to dating and relationships.

Abnormally Funny People

In 2004, I was working with Sky Television, training their contact centre staff and helping with the wording describing television shows for their Electronic Programme Guide. Sky Television was leading the way in including disabled customers, as were their other projects such as creating a more accessible physical remote control.

I encouraged them to go beyond subscribers and look at the representation of disability on television: they were a broadcaster. They explained that for them, there was a difficulty. Sky did not make any shows; they bought them already formed and broadcast them. They had little or no influence on the content of the shows, just whether they would buy it or not.

My contact was a tour-de-force called Kay Allen. She asked me, 'How can we make a TV show which has disability in it?' My reply was that I felt comedy and disability was a genre that could be interesting and needed change. I felt disabled people, comedians and writers should create and perform the comedy and take ownership. I felt disabled-led comedy in the form of stand-up was almost invisible. A few individual disabled comedians were working hard but low profile and on their own.

Knowing my dislike of how comedy has used dwarfism, this was a calculated gamble. Not exactly 'the best form of defence is attack', but there was something about taking control, leadership and breaking our own boundaries. There was an underlying ambition too: I had always wanted to perform stand-up comedy.

My suggestion was to bring a team of comedians together, all disabled bar one. The non-disabled one would be Steve Best, a best friend from school and a professional comedian. He would be our 'token' non-disabled one. Steve and I would create, perform and produce the comedy show at the Edinburgh Festival Fringe which, in case you don't know, is epic. Comedians refer to it as just 'Edinburgh', and it is the world's largest performance arts festival. Every August, tens of thousands of performers perform in thousands of shows in a myriad of venues. If you wish, you can see a show every hour from 11 a.m. to 1 a.m. every day. The Fringe has been where many now famous comedians cut their teeth. I thought doing our show every day, making people laugh alongside other disabled people, would be great. A disabled-led show with disabled comedians in a mainstream venue at a world famous arts festival would be groundbreaking. And Sky could make a documentary of us creating the show and then film the show itself. It would be two television shows from one project. Kay liked it, and green-lit it.

I asked Steve Best, the non-disabled professional comedian, to help. I had the vision, he knew the industry, I knew disability and he knew comedians. Finding the line-up was difficult. There were a few comedians who were disabled as mentioned and some others who happened to be disabled but did not talk about it. We realised we had to discriminate ourselves, to get a representative range of comedians and impairment types. After talking, searching, watching, we had our line-up. Liz Carr (wheelchair user) Tanyalee Davis (dwarfism) Steve Day (Deaf), Chris McCausland (blind) and Steve Best (not disabled) and me. We brought in a hugely experienced comedy director in Huw Thomas and set about creating the show.

There were hurdles. One act was relatively new to acquiring a disability and felt uncomfortable with the focus on it. Were we over emphasising it? Did we risk voyeurism or being like a circus show? I am not sure he ever truly overcame this concern during the run, but now, he is ok. We were happy as he was a fantastic comedian.

We had two stipulations – the comedian did need to acknowledge the disability, if only for the reason that this was a disability-led show and the audience would spend time wondering what the disability was! The second stipulation was on language and representation. The comedians could mock themselves, other disabled people, the public, etc. but not be cruel or bullying.

My biggest fear was not about this not being a hit. I felt it in my bones that it would prove successful. My fear was about what might happen after. Would we accidentally give permission for non-disabled people to make jokes about disability? Would our freedom with our language, our irreverent take on disabled life, backfire? Would other disabled people, specifically those with dwarfism, be angry? Would the public get it? My fears did not materialise, not in any substantial way. One night, after the show finished, I sought the feedback of a respected disability campaigner. He said 'I've waited 20 years to see this. This will change the game'.

An important and unusual aspect of Abnormally Funny People is that it is still here. Many disability projects and schemes are created, flourish then fade to dust. After our initial run in 2005, I suggested to Steve we had to keep this alive. In the years that followed, it sometimes was a fun side project, a creative outlet that earned everyone extra money too. Other times, it was a labour of love. We have now performed two runs at the Edinburgh Fringe Festival and numerous other shows around the United Kingdom in Manchester and Brighton and internationally in Germany, Ukraine and the United States. We created a podcast and had numerous residencies at the Soho Theatre in London. We were approached by the Royal Festival Hall to do a show during the COVID lockdown in 2021. For this show, we pulled the whole team together and performed a 2-hour extravaganza with stand-up, sketches and songs. Five hundred people bought a ticket, and 400 stayed the distance, which for a Zoom show is pretty good. I had decided before the show, this would be the final ever Abnormally Funny People show. We would go out on a high. Because of the high, the joy and appreciation, I thought, maybe we should keep going.

Thankfully, Abnormally Funny People still get asked to perform. We may not promote ourselves, but people want to see our shows and comedians want to be part of it. I love it when we find new comedians and ask if they want to join and they do. Fabulous comedians like Rosie Jones, Lost Voice Guy, Tim Renkow, Don Biswas and Juliette Burton are just a few who we have reached out to or they to us and have become part of the team.

Steve officially stepped away in 2016 but then rejoins for one off projects. I still think, maybe we will wind it down but then someone will ask us to do something, or a good idea pops up and we reassemble and have fun and create fun.

> It is hard to put a leash on a dog once you've put a crown on its head. (Tyrion Lannister, Game of Thrones, Season 2, Episode 7: A Man Without Honor)

Did we change the game? It is hard to quantify. I sometimes look at who is where now – Liz Carr is a star of both television and stage. Chris McCausland is a regular on TV and has sold out UK tours. Tanyalee Davis has had numerous television appearances, returned to the United States and has cultivated a TikTok following of 3.2m people. Steve Day is a successful stand-up supporting big name comedians. Steve Best, our token non-disabled person, has left stand-up and now is a photographer, mostly of comedians. I am doing ok being me.

Another way to view the reach of Abnormally Funny People is to see what disability and comedy have appeared since. As a reminder, disability comedy on TV is mostly patronising or simply avoided. Unlike comedy and dwarfism, there was a hesitancy with comedy and disability. Shows that have appeared since, written by or including disabled actors and characters include the black comedy series *Jerk* (2019-present). Written and starring Tim Renkow, a stand-up with cerebral palsy and an occasional Abnormally Funny Person, it has had three hit series and is unique and blisteringly funny. Laurence Clark, a long-standing friend, comedian and sometimes producer with Abnormally Funny People, had a TV pilot of his self-penned show *Perfect show* broadcast in 2022. He is a writer for many television shows now. *The Last Leg* (2012-present), a long running, topical comedy show fronted by two disabled comedians and a non-disabled one, has had many guests from Abnormally Funny People. Rosie Jones is a growing comedy force in the United Kingdom right now and has had multiple television shows of her own. In 2018, Lost Voice Guy won the huge Britain's Got Talent. A comedian with cerebral palsy whose real name is Lee, did his first London gig with Abnormally Funny People at the Soho Theatre in 2012.

These comedians and actors are hugely talented. They most likely would have 'made it' anyway. That said, it is good to know there was a place where they could perform with other disabled people. It was a safe space, as we were all supportive of one another. It is good to have creativity and risk taking space as we can play with disability and how people think about it, then perform it on stage.

> Never forget what you are, the rest of the world will not. Wear it like armour and it can never be used to hurt you. (Tyrion Lannister, Game of Thrones, Season 1, Episode 1: Winter is Coming)

Dwarfism and Comedy

I think when it comes to humour and dwarfism, there is an extra element. On *Family Guy*, they made a joke which I am quoting from memory saying 'Little people are God's gift to comedy'. This might be a difficult line for me to hear, but I do not see it as offensive in itself. It speaks a truth about lazy comedy writing, i.e. the thought that if you 'use a dwarf', the scene will somehow become funny. *Family Guy* is progressive at shifting attitudes. They show their characters as flawed, ignorant and biased. They highlight the viewer's ignorance or bias and throw it back out of the screen. They do not discriminate in which group of people to focus on. Instead, they manage to weave sexism, racism, ableism, ageism and other isms and phobias into the script, no one is off limits. They can make you laugh, sometimes awkwardly.

There has been progress on how we view dwarfism and disability, but I also see them as different. I think society mistakes 'supporting' disabled people, and it might come from a place of pity. They think it must be difficult to be disabled so associate it with tragedy or inspiration. But they do not feel sorry for people with dwarfism, for having dwarfism. It feels like it is something else. Is it not relatable? They can relate to being deaf, using a wheelchair and having depression, but not to dwarfism. They certainly cannot ever become it. Do they see it as a disability? Maybe people do not see it the same way as more 'classical impairments' such as mobility limitations or sensory loss.

Comedy about people like me can be complicated. Just because we have dwarfism, it does not mean we all have the same view. It is nuanced. One of the original Abnormally Funny People comedians is Tanyalee Davis who is short too and references it a lot in her comedy. She is an absolute barnstormer of a comedian, professional and top-notch. When she has a good gig, of which she has a lot, she will blow the roof off. As producers, Steve and I would get her to close a show because we knew she could do it. Mind you, when we did not get her to close, she was not happy. Yet, she is also the only comedian in my time as a producer that I have had to speak to about dwarfism jokes. As a producer, my philosophy is that comedians perform whatever material they choose, so long as it works and is funny. Their set can be about disability or dwarfism or not. But I did have to speak with Tanyalee. She was using the word 'midget' in one of her jokes. It is commonly agreed among the dwarfism community; it is an offensive word. I think one reason we do not like it is that it is never said neutrally – it is either part of a joke or as a term of abuse. We refer to it as the 'M word' to avoid saying it in full.

I explained to Tanyalee that when she is with Abnormally Funny People, she cannot use that word as it is offensive. She pushed back explaining she too is affected by dwarfism, so if she is ok with it, she should be able to. She has her own lived experience and view. She pushed back further, this time as a comedian, explaining it is a funnier word than 'dwarf' or 'little person' and gets a bigger reaction from the audience. My concern was people with dwarfism who came to see us would be offended. I was also concerned some non-disabled people would hear it and think it was acceptable language because someone who was directly affected was using it. I continued, if I had been an audience member, it would tarnish the whole show for me, and I did not want the public to think it is ok to say it.

Despite her push back, I held firm saying it is not negotiable. When she is part of Abnormally Funny Person, the word or whole joke goes. She has mountains of good material, so dropping one gag was not a problem. She is also pragmatic, realising the loss of work and future opportunities was greater than adjusting her set. She agreed and has not used it with us. At the time, in 2005, I think she had a point in the comedic sense. In 2023, I am curious to see if the audience would still laugh more at the M word. That said, I do not wish to try it and find out.

I have some control with how dwarfism is spoken about and how it is portrayed with Abnormally Funny People and our comedy. In another area, at the National Theatre as a board member, I do have a voice but I do not make artistic decisions as a board member. We had a Christmas show called *Hex*. Another brilliantly created and performed show, as is expected at the National Theatre. A take on Sleeping Beauty, Hex has a huge cast including a comedy troupe. In the troop of say 10 people, one had dwarfism. When they came on stage with everyone else, I flicked back to being 10 years old watching pantomime and wondered would I be wincing? Hex has had two runs at the National Theatre, and in the first run, the character delighted me, the second I was disappointed. There is a moment where the comedy troupe all move chaotically around the stage although they are choreographed movements. Second run of Hex, the character with dwarfism, started high kicking, so his foot reached his forehead. He continued to do this around the stage. My heart dropped. This was not great. This is for me, taking self-deprecation too far. My bet is the actors were asked to do something they wanted, be 'wild and wacky'. This actor, not realising his choice was demeaning, started doing this. The director presumably thought it is his choice so therefore ok.

In the first run of Hex, however, I was heartened. Same troupe, same chaotic movements. This time, it was creatively beautiful. The actor with dwarfism reaches out to a stooping average-sized actor. The short actor placed their hand on the other actor's forehead while their arms flayed around trying to reach the short person. If you have not recognised it already, it is the reverse of the cheap jokes of the 70s and 80s cruelly keeping someone with dwarfism at arm's length. I am not sure how many people in the audience noticed either the high kicks to the head or the reverse control arm reach. And if they did, did it make them think? I noticed both times, and it had a significant impact.

> When you tear out a man's tongue, you are not proving him to be a liar, you're only telling the world that you fear what he might say. (Tyrion Lannister, Martin, 1998)

Not for the first time I found myself judging someone else. Wishing to censor (or applaud) them is difficult territory. If the actor with dwarfism chooses to kick their own head, is it down to me to comment, to object? I might be a producer of Abnormally Funny People or a board member of the National Theatre, but should I be restricting this if a person like me chooses it? I know how I feel about it when it is bad, but I also feel conflicted because I am venturing into judging people's lives, people's work and what people choose to do.

The word 'choose' is important. It is a choice to sacrifice your dignity as no one with dwarfism is forced into entertainment. I do not have much time for the excuse some people use, as in 'I need to do this to pay the rent'. To demean themselves and demean everyone with dwarfism is a choice, not a necessity. I wince again when I think of those who dress up as a leprechaun and attend parties purely for the novelty value of their dwarfism. I wince at those who are thrown across a room for entertainment. I wince when someone is patted on the head or picked up for no reason. This is a choice. It is a choice to do something that takes very little skill or talent purely because of a genetic difference at birth. There are many jobs we can do and many other professions we do. I would still wince but give more respect if someone says 'I don't care and I like the money'. But making that choice impacts on all of us and continues the ridicule and ostracisation. It perpetuates the difficulties with identity and self-worth for some young people with dwarfism.

I do not like censoring people. I am fundamentally a liberal, so this makes it awkward for me. Being older and wiser and from experience, as strong as my feeling is, I hesitate when venturing into restricting individual freedom. I may fundamentally disagree with someone's choices; they might make my life more difficult, but I know they can be nice people.

A Life Lesson

Fresh out of university and politically fired up, I was part of a television documentary about a male stripping group called *The Half Monty*. The strippers were all people with dwarfism. I will admit it is a witty name, but that was the only thing I liked. I suggested a documentary to explore what the public felt when watching men with dwarfism (not trained strippers) taking their clothes off. I wanted to ask if this was an acceptable form of entertainment in modern society. I wanted to highlight the impact it can have on everyone else who has dwarfism. Despite the idea coming from me and agreed as a good one, the production ran away from the brief. During filming, it turned to ask why I was miserable. As I have already explained, the clichéd counter argument was used: being the stripper were earning income making the best out of their dwarfism and they were having fun. Here was educated, privileged Simon trying to stop others from doing what they wanted.

The documentary producers suggested I went to see *The Half Monty* live, so I could make a more informed comment. I took their point, but I already knew what it would be like and it was. Poorly trained, messy on stage and lacking talent, the public laughed at them, not with them. At times, they were picked up or patted on the head. There was a surface level sense of fun maybe but I sensed a deep sadness, a loss of dignity about the show. This was not a comfortable space for me; I knew some of the strippers which amplified the tension. I watched the show in a nightclub in the Midlands and was interviewed on film straight after. I became upset as the questions suggested the show was great; I was the problem. I remember welling up realising the premise of the documentary was slipping away and the producers showed lazy ignorance. They only saw people making choices and not the impact those choices made. The final broadcast documentary had probably 24 minutes of the strippers laughing while being patronised. I appeared for a couple of minutes, upset, poorly lit, utterly alone and unsupported. I said on film 'This doesn't feel right, and there are consequences', but the imbalance of me compared to the strippers was huge.

As is often the way with shows about disability, it was picked out by television reviewers in the press. Known for being highly opinionated critics, Victor Lewis Smith and AA Gill thankfully saw the bias in the documentary and recognised my point. They too asked why this was considered acceptable entertainment. It was a sort of win. Because of the experience, I decided from then on, rather than spending time and energy being critical of others; I would support the progressive and interesting representation and work to counter the demeaning. Eventually, the good work would dwarf the demeaning. Yep, that was deliberate.

> Death is so final. Whereas life, ah, life is full of possibilities.
> (Tyrion Lannister, Game of Thrones, Season 1 Episode 2: The Kingsroad)

The impact of demeaning people with dwarfism, for us forever being on trial has at its most extreme, led to some taking their own lives. Maybe there are some other reasons, but I know repeated jokes and demeaning dehumanising depictions of yourself do not help. Social media needs work and is not balanced. There is still ridicule of people with dwarfism, and it pops up regularly on my feeds uninvited. My work is not to ban certain roles. I have considered opinions, but it is not me who decides what the limits are. I want to continue to improve how people with dwarfism appear through all forms of media so the good stuff (in my eyes) becomes the dominant one. My work has been to enable people to understand some treatment of people with dwarfism is horrific and damaging. It is to make the world understand that we have a physical disability like someone who uses a wheelchair, who you would not dream of demeaning in the same way.

> It is easy to confuse 'what is' with 'what ought to be,' especially when 'what is' has worked out in your favour. (Tyrion Lannister, Games of Thrones, Season 5, Episode 9: The Dance of Dragons)

There is a serendipity about me joining Channel 4's *Gogglebox*. I have spent 20 plus years trying to change the representation of people with dwarfism and other disabilities on television or on stage. I have supported the talented disabled people, and I have advised the creative makers to make more representative and better shows. I have been behind the scenes, mostly. When *Gogglebox* came calling, it felt like an opportunity to be on screen in exactly the way I wanted dwarfism to be seen when I was a child. I liked the idea, the fun, the showing off. At the risk of sounding pompous, this was a chance for me to be the change I wanted to see.

My work is about the next generation of children with dwarfism. A friend has recently adopted a baby who has dwarfism. I want to know that this child's life will be full and interesting. The child will have some difficult moments but everyone does. Now, the amazing thing is when they watch television, go to the theatre, read a book or something else; they are less likely to see someone like them being ridiculed based purely on their physical height. The child is more likely to see someone with dwarfism just being themselves, a participating and respected part of society compared to 30 years ago. This in turn means when they go out, they are less interesting, even boring so do not receive as much unwanted attention.

Have things changed for the better and for good? While talking with an established talent agent, we both agreed things are better for disabled people and people with dwarfism in entertainment, be it opportunities, inclusion, access and more. I confessed to worrying it might cause another flash in the pan. She replied, 'No, It is changed, It is here. If anything, we're embarrassed about how long It is taken us to do this'.

Does that mean no more wincing for me? Undoubtedly. Now, it is more likely to be 98% joy and 2% sadness. I feel deep joy when I think of two young British actors with dwarfism. Lenny Rush, who is 14 and has the same condition as me and Fran Mills who is mid 20s and has achondroplasia. Their stage and screen careers are stratospheric. The roles they are offered, the roles they take, are brilliant. However, it has taken a long time, and I know a super talented person born with dwarfism who is roughly my age. She turned her back on performing as she believed she would never get a decent role. She now has a good job and good life, but the world did not get to see her perform. It is taken a while for the entertainment industry to see us as a whole human.

References

A Man Without Honor. (2016). *Game of Thrones*, Season 02, Episode 07. Directed by David Nutter. Written by David Benioff and D. B. Weiss. First broadcast 1st May 2016 [DVD]. Burbank, Warner Brothers.

Living in Oblivion. (1995). Tom DiCillo [film] Sony Pictures Classic.

Martin, G. R. R. (1998). *A song of ice and fire: A clash of kings*. Harper Collins.

Mostly Media. (2023). 10 years of Gogglebox [online]. https://mostlymedia.co.uk/10-years-of-gogglebox/#:~:text=At%20its%20peak%20during%20the,third%20most%20viewed%20scripted%20show. Accessed on November 29, 2023.

Oathbreaker. (2016). *Game of Thrones*, Season 06, Episode 03. Directed by Daniel Sackheim. Written by David Benioff and D. B. Weiss. First broadcast 8th May 2016 [DVD]. Burbank, Warner Brothers.

The Dance of Dragons. (2015). *Game of Thrones*, Season 5, Episode 9. Directed by David Nutter. Written by David Benioff and D. B. Weiss. First broadcast 7th June 2015 [DVD]. Burbank, Warner Brothers.

The Laws of Gods and Men. (2014). *Game of Thrones*, Season 4, Episode 36. Directed by Alik Sakharov. Written by Bryan Cogman. First broadcast 11th May 2014 [DVD]. Burbank, Warner Brothers.

The North Remembers. (2012). *Game of Thrones*, Season 2, Episode 1. Directed by Alan Taylor. Written by David Benioff and D. B. Weiss. First broadcast 1st April 2021 (DVD). Burbank, Warner Brothers.

The Station Agent. (2003). Tom McCarthy [film] Miramax Films.

Winter is Coming. (2011). *Game of Thrones*, Season 01, Episode 01. Directed by Tim Van Patten. Written by David Benioff and D. B. Weiss. First broadcast 17th April 2011 (DVD). Burbank, Warner Brothers.

Chapter 8

Creating Our Own Path: The Easterseals Disability Film Challenge

Nic Novicki (Creator of Easterseals Disability Film Challenge)
USA

Erin Pritchard (Senior Lecturer in Disability Studies)
Liverpool Hope University, UK

Introduction

I have been very lucky in my career. I have been in over 40 TV shows and movies. I have had the opportunity to work with Martin Scorsese and the Farley Brothers and tour all over the world as a comedian. Most recently, I was in *Spider-Man: Across the Spider-Verse* (2023), where I play Lego Spiderman. The majority of my work has been self-driven with me writing, producing and creating my own content. When I started getting into acting, I was getting some opportunities but not really the opportunities that I was very excited about, such as the love interest or the gangster. Those were not coming to me through traditional auditions.

Over a decade ago, I asked myself the question, 'Why aren't more people with disabilities creating their own content?' Approximately, one in four Americans identify as having a disability (Centers for Disease Control and Prevention, 2023). Those numbers translate worldwide. Disabled people are the largest minority population in the world (Baldev, 2020). The Annenberg Inclusion Initiative at the University of Southern California found that in 2022, only 1.9% of all speaking characters in the most popular movies of 2022 had a disability (Smith et al., 2023).

I started to produce my own content, such as short films and web series. Then I started to produce independent films. After that I created a whole body of work where I was showcasing myself in the roles that were the best way to represent myself as an actor and things that I was very proud of and also market myself in a different way as an actor which led specifically to jobs. It opened up the door for me, working with other independent producers and directors and casting directors.

Easterseals Disability Film Challenge

I did not want to be in a static place of representation. Little people and other people with disabilities cannot wait for the opportunities to come to us. As a result, in 2014, I launched the Disability Film Challenge. It is a 5-day film-making competition where you have to have somebody with a disability in front of or behind the camera. At first, I thought it was just going to be a one-off competition to help some friends with disabilities to create opportunities for themselves as well as get the opportunity to be showcased by the industry. In the first year, we only had about five films, and some of those films were created by little people as well as people with other disabilities. We put all those films online, and all of a sudden, casting directors around the world started contacting me and saying, 'Hey, how could we get in touch with this person or that girl, or this guy or who wrote this?'

In 2017, I partnered with Easterseals in Southern California. Easterseals is the United States' largest disability services organisation. It is a non-profit organisation that started in 1919 to support disabled people. Now, the challenge is called the Easterseals Disability Film Challenge. Easterseals bolsters the representation of the Disability Film Challenge, using its numerous communications channels to encourage participation. Year after year, the challenge has grown and attracted more people with disabilities. It allows them to take their career in their own hands and make films that showcase them exactly how they want to be showcased.

I have been very proud that the challenge has grown significantly. In over a decade, we have had over 600 films created from around the world. It is people with disabilities, including disabled actors, writers, producers, directors and film-makers that are telling their stories and getting opportunities in front of them behind the camera. I am very proud that so many little people have been a part of it throughout the year, and it has also given them the ability to announce themselves as being a part of the disability community.

The process starts with people registering. Our registration opens at the Sundance Film Festival in January, and every year, our challenge is in April. Those registered will receive the full assignment which includes themes, props and locations to choose from. While the contributors all know what the genre is, they do not know the full assignment until the start of the challenge. At the start of that five-day film-making challenge, I send out sub themes, props and locations for people to choose from. This ensures that these films are done over the course of five days, making it equitable for all people whether they have full cast and crews and all kinds of fancy camera equipment or if they just have a camera phone. They still have the ability to create a film and tell their stories.

Everybody goes to our website, which is at disabilityfilmchallenge.com, to firstly register and then check out the annual genre. We have done documentary, romance, sci-fi and buddy comedy. The latter which is what all of our alumni selected this year. A buddy comedy is based on two friends, who usually have contrasting personalities, who go on a mission or an adventure. Examples include *Stir Crazy* (1980), *Trading Places* (1983) and *Planes, Trains & Automobiles* (1987).

Every film has to have one person with a disability in front of or behind the camera, but some films end up having as many as a dozen people with disabilities. We have had even 20 people with different disabilities, from little people to those with invisible disabilities. I think it is very important for disabled creators and actors to not only be in front of the camera but also to be behind the camera because frankly, there are more employment opportunities behind the camera than there are in front of the camera. There are opportunities to be an editor, a script coordinator, a writer, a producer, a director, an assistant director or a producer. These roles enable disabled people to be in a position of power. They are part of the story and are a part of shaping the story and the narrative as a producer or as a writer. This allows you to be able to make sure that the story and what you are telling is done authentically.

In 2023, we had a record-breaking 115 films that were created from around the world. Everybody had the same assignment which was romance, but everybody had a different interpretation of that assignment and a different way for them to embrace their films and embrace who they are. I am proud of this authenticity that has come through the films. Even though it was romance last year, some films are really funny. Some films are really heartfelt, touching and dramatic. It is an interpretation of those individuals with disabilities. Sometimes, people do not even talk about their disability. They could just be a little person who is a bank robber, but he never addresses that he is a little person. Sometimes, it is good to include their disability, and they can talk about it in a subtle way or in a very obvious way. The fact that they are a little person or a wheelchair user or that they are blind, however, they want to, but they are able to do that through a narrative story, and sometimes, that is in a funny way or a scary way, depending on what the genre it is.

Little People and Comedy – Is It Ok to Laugh?

Little people have an uneasy relationship with comedy. Throughout history, people with dwarfism have been represented as figures of fun and usually the butt of the joke (Pritchard, 2021). In most cases, characters with dwarfism in films and television shows are laughed *at*, but rarely *with*. But, that does not have to be the case. Throughout my career as an actor and comedian, I think times have changed in a much greater way, in terms of better representation of the disability community and specifically the little people community. Throughout my professional career, there have been times where I have been hired as an actor, and whether it be for comedy or a dramatic scene, I have suggested to the writers and the directors that when a joke comes to play that instead of me being the joke, I am in on the joke or I am part of the joke.

I think we do need to be conscious of making sure that disabled actors and specifically little people actors can be part of comedies. We want to avoid a situation where people are scared to include us because they are going to do it wrong. I think the best way to do it right, or authentically, is when you have people with disabilities involved in the writing room and involved in the producing group. I have seen throughout my career that people are open to feedback. Comedy and really modern storytelling is about dialogue and exchanging ideas. I think that there are times that people can make a joke that involves me and me being a little person and that it is acceptable if it is done the right way, and my character is a part of it and it is justified. Also, if my character were to say something back and respond and educate. We can educate in subtle ways through comedy.

My background is in stand-up comedy. I started giving speeches when I was 8 years old raising money for Little People of America. I would always open up a lot of times with a joke. In some places I performed, there would be a podium and they would forget a stool. I would open up and say, 'Hey, you guys do you guys remember the stool? Or who will plan this?' I would do it humorously and let the organisers and audiences know that I am okay with the situation. I would have fun with the situation. I would use humour to break the ice and prompt them to make sure that in the future, there is a stool or a hand-held microphone. I realised that by opening with a joke, I was able to break the ice and get everybody's attention because comedy can get people to listen. When you stand up there and lecture people about what they are doing wrong, that is very important but I think when somebody is doing it through comedy that can grab the audience's attention.

Reaching Out and Getting Recognised

The goal of the Easterseals Disability Film Challenge is to create opportunities for disabled actors, writers, directors and producers in front of and behind the camera, but it is also to change the way the world views disabilities through these films. These films do not exist just within a film festival. All the films end up on our social media pages, including YouTube, Instagram and Facebook. We leave it up to each individual and film team to come up with their own campaign for their film to promote themselves. So not only are they making films, but we have an awareness campaign where each individual and film-maker tries to get as many likes, views and shares for their films. It encourages them to not only make the films but also to get themselves and the stories out there.

The film challenge enables people with disabilities to be discovered by networks and studios, and casting directors find them telling their stories in a very authentic way. We have casting directors, producers and executives who see all of these amazing films, and it reaches them through different channels, whether that be a news piece about the challenge or through the awareness campaign. The film challenge has given exposure to executive producers and casting directors where they have been able to see these stories but also to meet actors with disabilities, including little people. It allows them to not only see the work but also think about having more little people involved in a film.

When a little person who has made a film for the Easterseals Disability Film Festival and it ends up winning, or it ends up getting press, or it ends up getting turned into a bigger project that leads to more opportunities for them. It also leads to more opportunities for executives, cast directors and producers to advocate for that little person. It is a toolset that is marketable and that can be shared. If they are able to see a little person as the lead, they are able to see what that would look like if a little person were in a position of power, of being a boss, of being a villain, of being a love interest, of being whatever they have decided to be. It gives writers and producers the tools where they cannot only just think in theory, but they can see them in action. I think that the way forward is to let us not just talk about what we want but let us be a part of creating that change, whether that is through the film challenge or whether that is through continuing to make independent films or short films.

I feel very proud of the impact that the Easterseals Disability Film Challenge has made in the fact that we have gotten a lot of people, jobs and opportunities. One example is a little person named Sofiya Cheyenne. She is a very talented actor. Sofyia entered the Easterseals Disability Film Challenge numerous times. She made a film called *Europe* in 2018, and as a result, Peter Farley created a recurring role for a little person actor. Farley came to the challenge because he is a mentor. We have a lot of mentors who are executives, writers, directors and/or producers that mentor the winners. Farley has been a part of the challenge and a huge advocate since the second year it started. He reached out to me and said, 'I have this recurring role, and I'd like to cast a little person actress in this. Do you have any ideas?' I was able to share 10 films from the challenge, which starred little people. Farley was able to review all those films and watch them and assess the acting ability of those in them and judge their suitability for the role he wanted someone to fulfil. Farley invited Sofyia to audition, and she got cast as Louise in *Loudermilk* (2018–2020), which is a television show on Netflix. This was Sofyia's first major role and first recurring role, and that all came from the challenge. I want to see more and more opportunities like that.

In terms of the future, I would like to see more and more television shows and feature films green-lit by studios and by networks that come from the challenge.[1] That is something that we are very excited about. It is trying to really encourage people to continue to take their short films and to develop them into episodic series, into feature films, and to do as much as they can to put them into a position where they can be green-lit.

References

Baldev, N. (2020). The world's largest minority. *Opportunity International* [online]. https://www.opportunity.org.uk/news/blog/the-worlds-largest-minority. Accessed on February 08, 2024.

---

[1] Green-lit refers to providing financial backing to a film pitch.

Centers for Disease Control and Prevention. (2023). *Disability and health data system (DHDS)* [online]. http://dhds.cdc.gov. Accessed on February 08, 2024.

Pritchard, E. (2021). "She finds people like you hilarious!" Why do we laugh at people with dwarfism? *Journal of Literary & Cultural Disability Studies, 15*(4), 455–470.

Smith, S., Pieper, K., & Wheeler, S. (2023). *Inequality in 1,600 popular films: Examining portrayals of gender, race/ethnicity, LGBTQ+ & disability from 2007 to 2022.* USC Annenberg Inclusion Initiative.

Chapter 9

Dwarfism Advocacy: A Life Tenure

Angela Muir Van Etten (Former President of Little People of America)

Introduction

As a dwarf with Larsen's syndrome, my self-advocacy began as a young child calling out to friends to slow down and wait for me and continues as an adult closing in on 70 years. This chapter starts with my developmental years in institutional care, at home and school. I attribute this solid foundation as fine preparation for law school and a 40-year law career combating negative stereotypes and discrimination for myself and others.

After overcoming employment discrimination as a law school graduate in both New Zealand and the United States, I highlight the range of law jobs I held over the years – barrister and solicitor, legal writer and editor, advocacy specialist. This chapter demonstrates how each position refined my disability advocacy skills. A review of how to advocate against negative encounters with the public is presented with the underlying premise that dwarfs are equal contributing members of society who should be accepted as such. My 40-inch (101 cm) height does not justify being raised up onto a pedestal or put down by pity, patronisation, ridicule or rejection.

A discussion of systems advocacy against dwarf tossing and architectural barriers in the built environment is presented within a framework of effective advocacy principles that can be applied to any situation. This chapter shows that advocacy makes change possible when people care enough to do something, commit to the cause for as long as it takes, collaborate and form coalitions with like-minded people, communicate with honesty and respect and, in my personal view, have confidence in God's ability to change hearts and minds.

Because people with dwarfism – like any class of people – are not all cut with the same cloth, the terms *dwarf, little person, restricted growth or short-statured* are all in play. Likewise, person-first (person with dwarfism) or identity-first (dwarf) language is a personal preference. It is not a case of right or wrong. Rather it depends on the person and sometimes the culture, which term is preferred.

In deference to individual language preferences, this chapter uses the terms interchangeably. Personally, I'm comfortable with all these terms but tend not to use short-statured to describe myself. I consider short stature to be a euphemism and inadequate description of dwarfism which is a medical condition involving much more than height. For instance, dwarfism can also involve impairments related to vision, hearing, orthopaedics and neurology, to name a few. And people who are short for no medical reason don't experience the same discrimination as people with dwarfism.

Developmental Years

My life began with grim predictions of an early demise. But after 2 years of institutional medical care, my parents brought me home to join my new-born baby brother. Common sense was the primary source of their wisdom. They expected the same from me as my average-size siblings – obedience, chores and good grades. From the outset they recognised, I needed discipline in the same way any child does. Unfortunately, not everybody understood this need. My mother recalls the day she was shopping with my brother and me. We shared a stroller and were told to stay put while she went into the store. I was 4 years old and fully capable of obeying instructions. But like typical children, we were not worthy of our mother's trust, and as soon as she turned her back, we both climbed out. Mom returned to find us running around and promptly spanked us both. An elderly gentleman on the street reprimanded her for disciplining me. How dare she hit a child so small? Brushing off his scolding, my mother retorted, 'The child is old enough to know exactly what she's doing!'

Many people were like the old man and did not hold me accountable for my actions. Some relatives spoiled me and growled at my parents for being too harsh on 'poor little Angela'. Thankfully, my mother offset any favouritism, especially from elderly aunts who regularly gave me more money than my brother and sister. When driving home from our visits, mom insisted that I share the extra with my siblings. My parents accepted me and taught me to accept myself. They helped me to reject the opinion of those who stared and made fun of me. I was taught:

> It's better to smile than scowl. After all, most people are only acting in ignorance and don't even realise they're being rude.

Independence was instilled in me. It was never assumed I couldn't do things. If something seemed too tough, I was encouraged to find a way of doing it. Stools made lots of things possible. Coat hangers were not only used for hanging clothes but also to flick light switches on and off and remove socks. The rail on one side of the wardrobe was lowered for me to hang my clothes up; the other side was left at regular height for my average-sized sister. My size was never allowed as an excuse to get out of anything. I worked at the kitchen counter standing on a stool and ironed using our adjustable height ironing board. I was included in family activities. For example, in mom's quest for me to have fun like the other kids at the beach, she hoisted me onto a handheld surfboard for a fast ride. However, her plan was upended when I was dumped onto the sand by three waves piled on top of each other. My board went flying, my bathing cap swished off and I rode in on the bottom of the ocean floor with my feet facing their soles to the sun.

My spiritual education began when I was seven years old. One night on a family vacation, we stopped to listen to street music. Open Air Campaigners were singing gospel songs and preaching about Jesus Christ's sacrificial love. When an invitation to receive His love and forgiveness was extended to the gathering crowd, I responded. I knew that I needed Jesus in my life. Ever since that night, I have known God's love and drawn on His strength and wisdom to get me through every circumstance. My parents did not protect me by keeping me out of school or sending me to a school for 'crippled' children. At age four, I began regular kindergarten. There was no reason not to. My size didn't affect my ability or intelligence, physical impairments could be accommodated and dealing with teasing children was something I needed to learn sooner rather than later.

In high school, there was one student I avoided like the plague. He was also a little person. Whenever his friends saw me, they would chant riotously and push him towards me, 'Here she comes, here comes your girlfriend. Go on, kiss her, she's just right for you'. That was all I ever heard, as I would disappear long before there was any chance of a successful thrust. At no time in our two years at the same school did we ever speak to each other. Our only communication was mutual recognition of the other's embarrassment. But why? As teenage little people, neither one of us was mature enough to reject the stereotype that dwarfs are destined to date one another.[1]

I always knew I would be something when I grew up and was exasperated to meet people who had their doubts about my future. Take, for example, the doctor I met when I was 14. He even asked if I went to school. He was one of those who didn't expect me to do anything as an adult. In contrast, my parents realistically pointed out that I would not be able to do everything other kids did but stressed the need for me to concentrate on my education. I understood this, worked hard in school and qualified to attend university.

Legal Training and Career

My decision to study law at university was a process of elimination. Teaching and accounting didn't interest me, and I had no aptitude for science, engineering, geology or art. The legal profession never occurred to me until my aunt suggested it. I was considering journalism as a career and decided that law would serve as fine preparation. Yet after law school graduation, I did not pursue work as a law correspondent for a media outlet. Instead, I ventured into work in a law office.

My work as a barrister and solicitor in New Zealand was in a legal aid court practice advocating for clients in civil and criminal courts. My size was no barrier. Many prospective clients remembered me from the courthouse as the 'little lady lawyer'.[1] If clients who had never seen me asked if I was the lawyer, I answered with a

---

[1] 'Debunk Dwarfism Stereotypes'. *Angela Muir Van Etten blog*. 1 May, 2023. https://angelamuirvanetten.com/debunk-dwarfism-stereotypes/

simple 'Yes', asked how I could help them and invited them to take a seat next to my law degree certificate hanging on the office wall. When we started discussing their legal problem, they realised I talked and sounded like a lawyer, so my lack of inches was irrelevant. Any preconception that little people exist exclusively to entertain and amuse the public was also demolished.

My aspirations for writing came to fruition in the United States when for 17 years, I worked as a legal writer for two different organisations. For Thomson Reuters, I wrote disability civil rights and other law books for lawyers, and for the Christian Law Association (CLA), I wrote on religious liberty issues for non-lawyers. Neither employer had any qualms about my height, and both willingly accommodated me with accessible furniture. At Thomson Reuters, I had my own office and desk which made it reasonable to lower the desk to a height accessible to me. At CLA, I primarily worked from a home office, but when at the law office, I shared space. So instead of lowering a desk, an adjustable height chair with an attached footrest was provided.

My position as an Advocacy Specialist and Coordinator was for the Coalition for Independent Living Options – a non-profit organisation modelled after the Center for Independent Living (CIL) in Berkeley, California – exclusively serving the needs of people with disabilities. For 14 years, I advocated for individuals seeking: special education services, independent living, access to emergency services, voting rights, fair housing and financial assistance for home modifications, public transportation services and social security disability benefits. Each job served as a stepping stone to the next one built upon by my law degrees from the University of Auckland in New Zealand, the University of Maryland in Baltimore and admission to the bar in New Zealand, Ohio and New York. Likewise, my advocacy credentials were built one brick at a time starting with enrolment in first-year law classes.

At 18 years old, the photographer taking my student ID photo asked me to step up onto a stool to be in camera range. I could not get onto the stool alone, did not want him to lift me and was too timid to stop him. But by my second year, I was no longer too short for the camera. No, I had not grown in the interim, rather I realised that the environment is built by people for people; it is not our dictator. It was not for me to follow the camera but for the camera to follow me. This time, I rejected a lift from the photographer, had him remove the camera from the tripod and lower it to my level.

When I graduated from the University of Auckland in New Zealand with a Bachelor of Laws, I never dreamed that 7 years later, I would be sitting in a law school classroom in Baltimore, Maryland. But my decision to marry an American and emigrate from New Zealand to the United States made further study necessary. In order to practise law in the United States, I needed the American juris doctorate degree and a licence to practise law in each state where I worked as a lawyer.

My attendance at the University of Maryland School of Law gave me another opportunity to self-advocate. When the University only offered me one-third credit for my NZ law degree, I filed a petition for review with the admissions committee requesting the two-thirds credit permitted by the American Bar

Association. At the end of the review hearing, the committee member who appeared to have the greatest influence on the other members commented, 'Well, you do act like a lawyer'. Although I didn't get the two-thirds credit I wanted, the committee met me halfway and gave credit for half my NZ law degree.

My admission to the bar of the High Court of New Zealand in 1977 and the Supreme Court of Ohio in 1984 did not automatically open doors into the workforce in either country. Rather many doors slammed shut as prospective employers couldn't imagine a client having confidence in a 40-inch-tall (101 cm) lawyer. Thankfully, I had enough imagination for all of us. Disability nondiscrimination laws in the private sector were non-existent when I began my legal career. Hence, employers freely expressed flimsy excuses and abhorrent career advice:

- *You won't be able to appear in court because the legal robe will be too long!*
- *Judges won't wait for you to run up and down the stairs to get instructions from a client in custody in the tombs.*
- *Get a job in government service where you'll work behind closed doors and won't need to deal with the public.*

Some employers could not even discuss the possibility of me joining their staff. Their total shock at my appearance prevented them even giving me a hearing. I'll never forget a 'so-called' interview with one lawyer. He did no more than invite me into his office and offer a seat. He immediately accepted a phone call and 'eyed' me throughout his lengthy conversation. When the call ended, so did the interview.

At another interview, the attorney disrespectfully leaned back into his leather chair, put his feet on the desk and only asked questions unrelated to the job or my work experience. When he finally put his feet on the ground, I knew he was about to wrap the interview and was not considering me for the position. With nothing to lose, I challenged him for the questions he did not ask. This startled him into a bolt upright position followed by one open-ended query. My reply did not erase his prejudice, but at least he learned his bigotry was exposed.

Combating Negative Encounters

Although dwarfs are no longer 'sideshow' exhibits, we are still 'on show'. We are not billed as *Great Curiosities*, but we still arouse great curiosity and are still promoted as figures of entertainment (Pritchard, 2023). Fifty-five years ago, a Washington, D.C., attorney of 55 inches (139 cm) advised a teenage little person to take advantage of the attention. In his letter of encouragement, David Hornstein advised:

> Most people strive to be noticed. Don't pass it up. It is a motivator. You will do well while you're being noticed.

I wonder if Hornstein would give little people the same advice today. Would he see being ignored, stared at or filmed, disrespected and touched, questioned, verbally abused or ridiculed and discriminated against as a motivator? I doubt it, especially for negative encounters that escalate way beyond being noticed. So what advice do little people need today? As with many things, there is no one satisfactory answer. It totally depends on the situation, the little person's personality and sometimes even on how the little person feels on a particular day. So here is how I have handled various negative scenarios.

When customer service representatives ignore me, they may speak to the person in my company like I am not even there. For example, when arranging a seat assignment at an airline counter, the representative asked my friend whether I would like to sit next to the window. My friend knew better than to answer for me! I intervened. Even though I heard what the representative had said, I asked her to repeat and direct the question to me, the person who would be using the seat. That day, the representative received instructions that little people can speak for themselves. However, there is not much I can do in the moment when someone will not look at me, not even out of the corner of their eye or to sneak a peek when they think I am not looking. They completely deny my presence and remove any opportunity for us to communicate. An honest reaction is way better than being ignored.

An overwhelming majority of people with dwarfism suffer from strangers pointing fingers and piercing eyes that will not let go of their gaze (Pritchard, 2021; Shakespeare et al., 2010). The sight of someone so short is more than they can handle politely. I typically do not inflame the encounter with a frown and sometimes try to improve the situation with a smile. But for the most part, I take my parent's advice and ignore them. The 'take a picture it lasts longer' retort to someone staring at you is risky. The person could whip out their cell phone, snap a photo or take a video. This alarming trend is exacerbated by fears that the photos will appear on social media hate sites or as trophies on personal pages (See Ellis, 2018; Pritchard, 2023). Imploring shameless people not to click or post does not mean they will refrain.

According to one study, one-third of people with dwarfism have been physically touched by strangers in public (Shakespeare et al., 2010). We have been patted on the head for good luck, to see if we are real, or in the manner used to greet a child. Some even try to pick us up without permission. I inform such offenders that their behaviour is unwelcome and must stop. An invasion of my personal space is equally disrespectful. It happens when people discount my presence and encroach on the space immediately above my head. They might reach over my head to jump ahead at a check-out or serving line. Needless to say, the drip from a spoon passing overhead ignited my indignation when someone reached over me to get food from a buffet table.

The public often takes the liberty of asking personal questions. So many questions that I have an FAQ category on my weekly blog – *Angela Muir Van Etten blog: A voice for people with dwarfism & disability*. I write weekly blog posts as a tool for raising awareness, trying to change attitudes and behaviours and encouraging little people to become advocates. Questions like: Can you drive?

Why are you so short? Can I help you? Are you disabled? What should I call you? How old are you? Although it is easier to ignore questions, I have concluded it is in my best interest to answer most of the time.[2] When people say, 'I've never seen anyone as small as you', I know I am the inquirer's first contact with a little person. Typically, questions come without malice or intention to offend. If I do not increase their knowledge, they will go their way in ignorance and have a dim view of little people who rebuff their queries. However, I decline to answer obnoxious questions.

Not that I always get it right. For instance, I mistook the 'how old are you' question from a man old enough to know better as not worthy of an answer. I sarcastically asked him if he was planning to tell me how old he was. He apologised and explained that his grandson is a little person and he wondered if he would live to a good old age or if his lifespan would be as short as his height. I disclosed my 60 something age and explained that, in most cases, height does not correlate to age at either end of the spectrum. Of course, there are times when I will not answer genuine questions of polite people simply because I'm tired of my unpaid 'appointment' to public relations. Questions are shelved with a smile, and I move on. After all, a public relations volunteer cannot be on duty 24 hours a day, 365 days of the year.

Researchers report that three-quarters of people with dwarfism have been verbally abused (Shakespeare et al., 2010). Names like midget, hunchback and runt are derogatory and worthy of disdain. Short-stature synonyms like pint-size, shrimp or shorty are demeaning. Little people are tired of being the butt of jokes. We are not amused at being ridiculed because of our appearance. For example, when I saw a group of bullies laughing, pointing and mimicking the way I walk, I interrupted and instructed them to get it right and walk without bending their knees. They quickly learned that my way of walking is no joking matter.[3]

My 40 inches (101 cm) in height do not justify being denied equality by a pedestal or paternalism. Being a dwarf does not make me better or worse, more or

---

[2]'Can You Drive?' *Angela Muir Van Etten blog [online]*. 20 June 2022. https://angelamuirvanetten.com/can-you-drive/ 'Why Are You So Short? Is the Answer in the Genes?' *Angela Muir Van Etten blog [online]*. 21 November 2022. https://angelamuirvanetten.com/why-are-you-so-short-is-the-answer-in-the-genes/ 'Can I Help You?' *Angela Muir Van Etten blog [online]*. 6 June 2022. https://angelamuirvanetten.com/can-i-help-you/ 'Are You Disabled?' *Angela Muir Van Etten blog [online]*. 24 May 2021. https://angelamuirvanetten.com/are-you-disabled/ 'What Should I Call You?' *Angela Muir Van Etten blog [online]*. 2 November 2020. https://angelamuirvanetten.com/what-should-i-call-you/ 'How Old Are You?' *Angela Muir Van Etten blog [online]*. 24 August 2020. https://angelamuirvanetten.com/?s=How+Old+Are+You%3F

[3]For further discussion on negative encounters, go to: 'Renounce Common Discourtesy, PLEASE'. *Angela Muir Van Etten blog*. 21 March 2022. https://angelamuirvanetten.com/renounce-common-discourtesy-please/ 'Say No To Bullies'. *Angela Muir Van Etten blog*. 11 October 2021. https://angelamuirvanetten.com/say-no-to-bullies/ 'That's Not Funny'. *Angela Muir Van Etten blog*. 17 August 2020. https://angelamuirvanetten.com/thats-not-funny/

less equal. I only achieve equality when my size does not cause people to raise me up to superhero or put me down as someone needing special treatment. It is not courageous for me to get out of bed in the morning and engage in routine daily tasks. And I do not need looking after. Rather, I need a handshake not a handout and accommodations that level the playing field.

Sheer numbers make it impossible to reach everyone individually. As a result, I influence the public via my blog, books, presentations and the media.[4,5] Opportunities abound in schools and businesses for disability sensitivity training to instil proper behaviours when encountering people with dwarfism. Student feedback after training gives me hope for more positive encounters in the future.

> The presentation was very eye opening and gave me a different perspective on everything. I've learned to be politically correct when involved with little people.
>
> I loved the stories you told us about your life and for clearing up things people will never understand from your perspective. I will never forget what you told us and will try to use that information.
>
> Hearing your lecture will be on my mind for the rest of my life.
>
> When you told me it is not disrespectful to sit down and talk to you and see eye-to-eye, I was shocked.

The media are attracted to little people. But ensuring that coverage is positive involves considering the reputation of the outlet before being interviewed. If I do not believe my message will be fairly presented, I decline the interview. This does not mean I avoid forums with an opposing viewpoint; rather I steer clear of outlets inclined to sensationalism and erroneous reporting. It is critical, therefore, for my interviews to identify negative encounters and invite positive interactions. For instance, I initiate content on 'four-letter words' that insult – abnormal, afflicted, burden, defect, midget and victim. In distinguishing size from equality, I stress our similarities and abilities. It is better to discuss how we're alike and what people with dwarfism can do. This advances our goal of being integrated and accepted as equal members of society. Moreover, our message will have a greater impact if we stand together. We will attract more attention and should take advantage of the ready-made audience waiting with their pens and cameras.

> Two can accomplish much more than twice as much as one,
> for the results can be much better. . .
> and one standing alone can be attacked and defeated,

---

[4]'Dwarfism Sensitivity & Awareness'. *Angela Muir Van Etten blog [online]*. 24 October 2022. https://angelamuirvanetten.com/dwarfism-sensitivity–awareness/

[5]'Tips for Achieving Positive Media Coverage'. *Angela Muir Van Etten blog [online]*. 27 February 2023. https://angelamuirvanetten.com/tips-for-achieving-positive-media-coverage/

but two can stand back-to-back and conquer:
three is even better,
for a triple braided cord is not easily broken.
~ Ecclesiastes 4:9, 12, Living Bible

Through the years, I have come to see my dwarfism as a gift that should not be wasted. I can use it to positively influence how people perceive disability, illustrate our abilities, interact with kindness, increase integration into the mainstream and identify barriers that demand removal. I can impede the impact of negative behaviours by being impervious to the impertinence, isolating offenders and indicting those who interfere with civil rights and impose inequality and injustice on people with disabilities.

Effective Advocacy Principles

When our sense of injustice is aroused to the boiling point, it spills over into action as we cry out: *Something has to be done about this!* Near the end of the 20th century, two monumental social injustices affecting the dwarfism community activated me: dwarf tossing and architectural barriers in the built environment. Dwarf-tossing spectacles masqueraded as 'sport' when barroom patrons in Florida and New York competed for prize money awarded to whoever threw a dwarf the farthest. A willing dwarf served as a human Frisbee when tossed into the air. And the foremost architectural barriers excluding people with dwarfism were the height of ATMs, fuel pump dispensers, point-of-sale terminals, soap dispensers, elevator buttons – everything activated with a push, pull or turn. In my quest for equal justice, I learned that commitment is personal. I cannot expect others to do something if I will not do anything. No one cares as much as I do.

In the case of dwarf tossing, I was compelled to stand against morally bankrupt behaviour that dehumanised and disregarded the value of little people made in the image of God, threatened little people with copycat bullies and encouraged the public to ridicule and discriminate against us. As a result, in July 1989, I was appointed as the Little People of America (LPA) Coordinator to promote a New York State law to ban this violent entertainment.

> This sort of struggle is personal for us. This is a blessing because it means that we fight that much harder than [ideologue politicians] do, but a curse because we feel the pain all the way down deep in our bones when we have to fight for our basic dignity as human beings. (Joe Stramondo, LPA Advocacy Director, 8 October 2011)

In the 1980s, a teenage little person complained in my LPA advocacy workshop about not being able to reach ATMs and asked, 'Who is going to do something about this?' At the time, I had no answer for her. But in 1994, I became 'the someone' when I agreed to be LPA's delegate on the ICC/American National Standards Institute (ANSI) A117.1 Committee on Accessible and Usable

Buildings & Facilities (ANSI Committee). LPA President Ruth Ricker offered me the position given my background as an attorney and advocate. When I hesitated, Ruth inquired, 'If you don't do it, Angela, who will?' Not finding anyone else lining up to tackle the giant, I saw the assignment as a calling from God.

It goes without saying that civil rights are invaluable and cannot be quantified. Nonetheless, before embarking on these campaigns, I weighed the personal cost in terms of time and money. I knew the toll would be heavy. For example, when coordinating passage of the New York State dwarf tossing ban, the commitment became burdensome when the legislative session coincided with my studying for and taking the New York State bar exam while holding down a full-time job. But God gave me the strength to do both, along with the prayer support of the women in my Bible study group.

As the LPA delegate on the ANSI Committee for seven years, I was constantly balancing the demands on my time at work and the physical strain of flying thousands of miles on the many trips between our residence in Rochester, New York and ANSI Committee meetings in Washington, D.C. I worked many Saturdays to earn compensatory time to attend meetings that lasted from one to three consecutive week days. Working on both dwarf tossing and environmental barriers drummed home that changing the world overnight was impossible. Dwarf tossing proved to be a perennial weed. No sooner would the weed be killed in one location, and it would pop up somewhere else. After a public outcry in Chicago caused contests to be cancelled in 1985, Philadelphia protests nixed contests in 1986. After the Florida legislature banned the practice in 1989, the promoters relocated to New York State.

Despite Florida's dwarf tossing ban, proponents resurfaced every decade or so. In November 2001, a Tampa radio personality, known as Dave the Dwarf, filed a lawsuit asking a federal court to find the law unconstitutional. (The case was dismissed.) In 2011, Florida State Representative Workman introduced a bill to repeal the ban declaring the law obsolete. (The bill died in Committee when the Florida legislative session ended in April 2012.)

Building code changes is incremental, and revisions are considered in five-year cycles. As a new delegate to the ANSI Committee, it would have been foolish to come out of the gate proposing amendments in every code section. Therefore, in the 1994–1998 cycle, I targeted the reach range provisions that regulated the height of anything activated with a push, pull or turn. LPA's proposed amendments related to lowering the unobstructed side reach from 54 to 48 inches. (Changes to eliminate the obstructed reach bathroom problems and exception for high-rise elevators with more than 16 openings were proposed in the 1998–2003 cycle.)

Choosing the right forum is key to effecting change. When negotiation and negative public reaction failed to stop dwarf tossing contests in Florida and New York, legislation was the only way to avert this throwback to freak show entertainment. But when promoters took the show on the road before municipalities could prohibit the practice with local ordinances, it became clear that the State legislature was the proper forum. A federal law was not called for because dwarf tossing was not a national problem.

LPA's attempt to remove the six-inch reach barrier on ATMs at the federal level initially seemed like the right move. After all, it was a national problem. But LPA's 1993 letter writing campaign to the Access Board did not convince this federal government agency to lower the unobstructed side reach from 54 to 48 inches in the federal Americans with Disabilities Act Accessibility Guidelines (ADAAG). But 1 year later, LPA learned that a better place to start was the ANSI Committee. ADAAG content was greatly influenced by the ANSI access code and agency staff who served on the Committee. And sure enough, 1 year after the ANSI Committee lowered the unobstructed side reach from 54 to 48 inches, the federal Access Board published a Notice of Proposed Rulemaking (NPRM) to update ADAAG with the same 48-inch reach standard. When the final rule was published on 23 July 2004, the six-inch reach barrier was broken and applied uniformly across the United States.

Competence is another big factor in effective advocacy. For example, learning and following the ANSI process was instrumental in gaining ANSI Committee member support. Observing the groaning and eye rolling at members who failed to follow procedure made this very clear to me. Earning respect on procedural matters gave me a fighting chance on substantive matters. It took skill to learn the facts and, on occasion, to generate the facts. In March 1995, when the majority of ANSI Committee members opposed LPA's proposed changes to the ANSI Access code, they cited the need for supporting statistical data. In the past, calls for research had been sufficient to ward off any moves for code revisions. Even though LPA did not have the requested data, we skilfully pulled the rug out from under those determined to keep the status quo. We launched a Measure-Up Campaign (reach range survey) at the July 1995 LPA national conference in Denver, Colorado, and produced data supporting the need for the six-inch reduction. Furthermore, it was also important to know ADAAG's amendment process. When the Access Board published the NPRM in 1999, I encouraged LPA's 6,500 members and other disability organisations to write letters supporting the federal rule change. The Access Board later reported that several hundred comments addressed the merits of lowering the unobstructed side-reach range to 48 inches, but only mentioned two organisations by name – LPA and the ANSI Committee, both of which I was privileged to have led to this historic change.

Effective advocacy involves making connections and building relationships with people on both sides of the issue. For example, my strategy of sitting next to different committee members at each ANSI Committee meeting allowed me to personalise the issue for those inclined to oppose any change to the reach range standard. Some were influenced to support LPA's amendments, but for those entrenched in their opposition, I listened to their objections and prepared counterarguments.

Building coalitions is an important component of effective advocacy. It involves constituents who share the same goal (other little people), allies who understand our issue (other disabled people) and supporters who care enough to help (family, friends and co-workers). For example, when coordinating the New York bill to ban dwarf tossing, my first step was to build a coalition of little people who shared my passion to stop the atrocity. On the ANSI Committee, I identified ANSI members in the disability membership category that LPA could rely on as allies to support our proposed amendments. The Disability Rights Education and Defense Fund (DREDF) was a powerful constituent for breaking the six-inch reach barrier. Little people and half a million people with various disabilities all benefited directly from LPA's proposed changes.

In forming coalitions, I learned the importance of coalition members pulling together. DREDF and LPA readily supported one another's proposed amendments. But access changes in bathrooms were a rare instance when the needs of our constituents diverged. Lower counters would provide sink (lavatory) access to little people but create barriers for wheelchair users. But instead of pulling against one another, we worked hard to find a solution that met the needs of constituents in both organisations. A satisfactory solution was achieved when industry consultants proposed leaving the sink at 34 inches (86 cm) for wheelchair users and installing faucets and soap dispensers within 11 inches (28 cm), the accessible forward reach of little people. This could be achieved with electronic activation or installation on the side rather than at the back of the sink. After following the many steps in the ANSI process, the proposal was approved as a revision to the 2003 ANSI Access standard.

One challenge with constituent coalitions is the contrary viewpoints within the ranks. For example, not all little people think LPA should advocate against dwarf tossing, especially those who are paid to be tossed. And we're all entitled to our own opinion. Likewise, we as activist little people are free to promote and defend a law that bans dwarf tossing. The content of campaign communications is critical. The message needs to be credible, consistent, convincing and confident. Credibility is lost when constituents exaggerate, such as claiming there are one million little people in America when it is more like 50,000. Consistency requires campaign representatives not to contradict one another. Convincing lawmakers may call for expert testimony. For example, the New York Assembly bill almost died in the Codes Committee because the proposed definition of dwarfism was too vague. Two members of LPA's Medical Advisory Board – Dr Cheryl Reid and Dr Charles I. Scott, Jr – were recruited to help committee staff draft text that precisely defined the people with dwarfism protected by the law.

Various communication platforms should be used – letters from constituents and disability allies; media reports, letters to the editor and blog posts; petitions; and meetings with legislators. LPA used all of these platforms in its campaign to convince Florida State Representative Workman to withdraw his repeal bill. He was ready to fold on 14 November 2011 when LPA turned up the temperature and delivered to his office 146 printed pages of a petition with 4,834 signatures from people in 49 states, Puerto Rico, the District of Columbia and 27 countries! The bottom line for successful advocacy campaigns is to follow the advice of Winston Churchill: 'Never give in; never, never, never, never'. And for me, I also counted on divine intervention based on perseverance, preparation and prayer.

Conclusion

If only there was a pretty bow to tie up this chapter. For as many advocacy victories we have to celebrate, there are so many more barriers to overcome. Where there are laws, we have non-compliance and enforcement issues. Where there are new technologies, we have design and funding failures that exclude people with dwarfism. Where there is inaccessible equipment, we have laws that stop short of mandating accessibility. In other words, we have a long way to go before we achieve equal access and respect. As a result, I have come to believe that as long as there are people living on this planet, there will be a demand for advocates. It is our job to train up people to follow in our footsteps teaching them that change is possible with preparation, perseverance, persuasion and prayer.

Be an advocate for positive change!

References

Ellis, L. (2018). Through a filtered lens: Unauthorized picture taking of people with dwarfism in public spaces. *Disability & Society*, *33*(2), 218–237.

Pritchard, E. (2021). *Dwarfism, spatiality and disabling experiences*. Routledge.

Pritchard, E. (2023). *Midgetism: The exploitation and discrimination of people with dwarfism*. Routledge.

Shakespeare, T., Thompson, S., & Wright, M. (2010). No laughing matter: Medical and social experiences of restricted growth. *Scandinavian Journal of Disability Research*, *12*(1), 19–31.

Chapter 10

Exploring Dwarfism Representation in Social Media: Intentionality and Advocacy as a Digital Content Creator

Kara B. Ayers (Associate Professor)

Cincinnati Children's Hospital Medical Center, USA

Introduction

The disability mantra, 'Nothing about us, without us', serves as a call to action for me and many disability advocates around the world. While our engagement in direct advocacy in person seems non-negotiable, it can be tempting to avoid the non-disabled online gaze and scrutiny through less engagement on social media platforms. In our absence on these platforms, however, the void is unfortunately filled with false assumptions, stereotypes and even mockery. Entering the foray of social media as a visibly disabled little person means facing society's stigmatising views and treatment of dwarfism head-on, especially related to our choices to reproduce. There are also benefits to online engagement, including access to other little people around the world and insights to make a largely inaccessible world more inhabitable.[1] All forms of dwarfism are considered rare conditions with just 1 in 10,000 live births resulting in a person with achondroplasia (Bacino, 2023) and 1 in 10,000–20,000 live births resulting in a person with Osteogenesis imperfecta (Balasubramanian, 2023). In a literal sense but more importantly, related to power dynamics of whose voice and stories matter, we are outnumbered. To achieve greater equity, we need our dwarf bodies, our dwarf perspectives and our dwarf experiences present in the same spaces where average-height (AH) people exist – often without question.

The social experiences and challenges associated with dwarfism can feel isolating, but social media has bridged our communities in ways not possible in the past. In a matter of moments, we can share an image, words or video with

---

[1] I will use the terms little person and dwarf interchangeably in acknowledgement that preferred terms vary by individual and community. Similarly, I will use both person-first and identity-first language approaches because both are valid ways to discuss dwarfism and disability.

someone else who has our rare condition. While the allure of connections within our community is strong, we are also sharing our images, identities and stories with non-disabled and AH people as part of the larger online social media landscape.[2] Some of these people are family members, friends and allies to the cause of anti-ableism, or pushing back on the idea that non-disabled or AH people are superior. Some of those who view our social media posts are notably not allies and may even use our posts to mock or cause harm. Just as little people are frequently photographed without their consent, their online photos are sometimes used to make insulting memes. This is but one of the many dangers of social media that digital creators must weigh against the multiple benefits of creating and sharing content that could dispel myths about dwarfism and prompt greater acceptance and inclusion.

The purpose of this chapter is to reflect on my experiences as a digital media creator with dwarfism who also researches the impact of disability portrayals in media. With the intention of self-reflexivity, or self-awareness of how my own biases, power dynamics and cultural backgrounds influence my interpretations, it is important to note that I hold both marginalised and privileged identities. I am a white, cisgender, female with Osteogenesis Imperfecta (OI), which is a collagen disorder and one of the approximately 400 types of dwarfism. Unlike some forms of dwarfism whereby short stature is the defining feature, the distinctive characteristic of OI is bones that break easily. Although I am four feet three inches (129 cm) tall, I did not identify as a little person until young adulthood. I had been a full-time wheelchair user since early childhood but as I began to traverse the world more independently, I began noticing the way height influenced my ability to access spaces and how I was perceived by others. It is through these lenses that I offer recommendations to prioritise quality over quantity of content to increase the representation of dwarfism in everyday life while also reducing ableism in media and beyond.

Personal Evolution as a Content Creator and Researcher

Background as a Content Creator With Dwarfism

While raising two teenagers and a school-age child who cannot wait to be a teen, I am reminded that growing up is hard! Even as a social media optimist, I am thankful that I did not have the same level of access to social media that many children have today. In addition to the typical dangers and complexities of navigating this form of online communication, my burgeoning identity as a young, disabled person would have undoubtedly been further complicated by this added layer. Young people with disabilities today must often navigate both the dangers and benefits of social media. My earliest introductions to what I perceived as dangers online related to exchanges from strangers who clearly seemed interested in physical aspects of my disabled body without knowing me as

---

[2]The term average-height people or AH people is a term used to describe people without dwarfism. It is acknowledged that some AH people have disabilities, demonstrating that discrimination faced by people with dwarfism also comes from other disabled people.

a person in any way. In the early days of the internet, chat rooms allowed people with disabilities to make direct and individual connections with others. These online gathering spaces were also frequented by devotees, people who fetishise disability and seek out images or items that represent disability to them in a sexualised way (Limoncin et al., 2014). I have always identified as disabled on my public online profiles.

Even as a teen, I viewed my disability as a part of who I was, and I yearned to connect to others who shared this identity. In addition to being contacted by other people with disabilities, I received unsolicited messages, often from adult men, requesting private information about my body or even pictures of the soles of my feet, which are apparently a hot commodity because I do not walk on them. While confusing, this was also my first introduction to the unique and specific need for people with disabilities to be aware and safe while communicating online. I came to realise that while I may not understand the motivations of others in soliciting information from me, they could use anything I shared in ways that could be harmful. I needed to be cautious about the ways that I shared information about myself online. As a disabled parent, I am aware of these dangers and can educate my disabled child but this specific risk of devotees targeting underage minors is often completely unknown to non-disabled parents.

My approach today to the intentional sharing of information online still resonates with a careful protection of private information that could be used to harm myself or my family. I am aware that people have varying motivations and can take statements, images or videos out of context and use them for their own purposes. At the same time, I have made life-changing connections through online interactions. Networked individualism emphasises the online connections and relationships that shape our identities and shift a social dynamic (Pritchard, 2021). In the digital space, we are not the extreme minority because even though I have a rare condition, I have found groups related to my type of dwarfism focused on a wide range of topics, including pregnancy, fashion, parenting and book clubs. I have found solidarity with other disabled people who seek similar goals and I have found that I am not alone in almost anything that I do. I have connected with world-renowned experts who are willing to share their knowledge and experience with me to troubleshoot or problem-solve a challenge that I have encountered as a little person with a disability. I have mentored dozens of people with disabilities, many from around the world, whom I would not have had the pleasure to know without our online connections, almost always forged first through social media.

My early forays into content creation as a digital artist with dwarfism date back to the days of Disaboom, an online blogging site for people with disabilities (Disaboom, n.d.). Disaboom was the largest social media platform for people with disabilities with more than 90,000 registered users (Apollo.io, n.d.). It was also among the first platforms to pay its writers with disabilities. It created a large database of reviews of public places based on users' perspectives about accessibility. Bloggers from this site became a community of their own. More than 15 years since the website closed its doors, I remain in contact with many of the bloggers. We wrote on a wide range of topics. I tended to focus on current events related to disability, advocacy efforts and what was top of mind at the time, my wedding planning! I reflect on these early writing days in all the simplicity of making decisions about what to share and what to maintain as private because the decisions were centred only on myself. When I write today, especially about my family or parenting, I also must consider the impact on my husband, our children and our family at large.

Several years after Disaboom closed, I became pregnant with our first child. I immediately recognised the lack of information available to parents with disabilities, and I sought to be a positive part of changing that problem. I created a small blog called 'Wheeler Mom' and began to write about my experiences with pregnancy and parenthood. Throughout my pregnancy and parenthood for my husband and I, the intersections of being little people and wheelchair users have been prominent aspects of what I share because I find them so absent in other representations across media. I transitioned to another blog called 'Roll You Home' a few years later as we pursued the adoption of my son from China. My son has achondroplasia, the most common form of dwarfism. He has never used a wheelchair and short stature is the most defining characteristic of his disability. For the blog about his adoption, I considered the multiple intersecting identities, especially those of which I held privilege, and my son did not. I wanted other parents with dwarfism who may be interested in adoption to learn from our process, so I was careful to share our experience with transparency while also respecting the privacy of my son's story, an important and valuable lesson I learnt by listening to many adult adoptees. Today I share our family's story, focused on my experience of motherhood, through posts to social media platforms, such as Instagram, Facebook, Twitter and TikTok. The transition to digital creation via social media instead of blogging has aligned with drops in the popularity of blogs and increased engagement across multiple social media platforms.

Journey as a Researcher Studying Disability Portrayals in the Media

Parallel to my path as a digital content creator, I have also studied the effects of disability portrayals in media through my role as a researcher. While not linear or complete, portrayals of dwarfism have at least somewhat evolved from freak show performances to a greater focus on education, pride and acceptance. Freak shows and circus-like performances have mostly ended but society still tends to view dwarfism as a form of amusement or entertainment (Pritchard, 2017). Society views dwarfism with humour and equates little people with non-human entities, like elves and leprechauns. These cultural representations have been shaped by the non-disabled, including AH people, because they largely control the media as a dominant majority. Some little people also contribute to these harmful stereotypes by agreeing to degrading performances that portray dwarfism and a non-human characteristic. Just as little people can contribute to harmful narratives, they can also add to positive or neutral portrayals. My research and advocacy aim to change the representation of dwarfism and other forms of disability in the media through greater direct engagement of media creators with dwarfism.

In addition to more accurate portrayals of dwarfism in the media, changing representation holds promise to bring down a wide range of barriers faced by people with dwarfism. Dwarfism is a visible disability and bodily difference. Goffman's (1963) stigma theory describes dwarfism as an ascribed stigma, recognising that a person is born with dwarfism, versus an achieved stigma, such as obesity, which people tend to judge more harshly because they believe people are responsible for their own condition (Backstrom, 2012). This variation in stigma can shift if people negatively judge the personal decision to have biological children as a person or people with dwarfism.

Many factors influence the reproductive decision-making of people with genetic disabilities that cause dwarfism. People with dwarfism are aware of stigmatising views about our decisions to reproduce. A doctor once told me, 'If I were you, I would adopt'. When I inquired if something about my health prompted this advice, the doctor clarified that he had made the statement based on his personal belief that he would not reproduce if he had an inheritable disability. It is not uncommon to see similar sentiments shared in comment sections announcing the pregnancy or birth of someone with dwarfism. Society's stigmatising views and treatment of people with dwarfism sometimes factor into highly personal decisions made by little people about whether they will have biological children.

The Intersection of Personal Experiences and Academic Pursuits

Much of my research has focused on the experiences of disabled parenting and pregnancy with a disability (Andrews & Ayers, 2016). Social support during pregnancy is important (Maharlouei, 2016), but many pregnant people with disabilities feel isolated and judged. Disabled mothers benefit from virtual communities hosted on social media platforms (Baker & Yang, 2018). These communities offer what many in-person networking opportunities cannot, a chance to connect with other disabled mothers and a chance to talk openly about pregnancy and parenting without stigma and judgement. My colleagues and I observed these benefits and co-founded *The Disabled Parenting Project*, a grassroots, community-based online support group, in 2016. The Disabled Parenting Project aims to connect disabled parents and also serves as a research community to better understand our experiences. I am both a contributor of content and a moderator for this community.

Sharing Glimpses Into Life as a Mother With Dwarfism

Intentionality Behind Sharing Personal Experiences

While the intended focus of my content as a digital creator is centred on my experience as a disabled person and mother, I cannot overlook the reality that sharing content about motherhood involves my children. Diverse representation and informed consent are both important to me but sometimes at odds. While I want to contribute to the lack of representation of mothers with dwarfism, sharing images – especially ones that feature vulnerability – of my children before they can offer informed consent sometimes comes at odds with my drive to protect them and respect their privacy. As my children have gotten older, it has become possible to acquire verbal consent to publish their images, but I am aware of the pressure they may feel to grant permission. We regularly share discussions about the permanency of the internet, their power to decide what images or stories are shared and how they might make their own decisions like this in the future.

Just as sharing our personal experiences as a family is a choice, so is not sharing. Sharing our images and stories is a concrete message to society, 'We are here'. Still, we are gatekeepers to many of our most cherished moments as a family. Non-disabled creators often encourage authenticity through sharing raw and vulnerable images. Disabled people are not afforded this privilege. As disabled parents, we risk additional scrutiny (Andrews & Ayers, 2016) that can even result in engagement with child protective services. When non-disabled parents post pictures of their children in distress, they are met with enormous outpourings of sympathy and support. Their children may be shown in compromising positions with little to no clothing or crying uncontrollably. I have coined this type of content as 'desperation porn' because it objectifies the subject (the child) for the gains (of sympathy) of the parent (Ayers & Reed, 2022). I do not share nor support the sharing of this type of content. There are other avenues for sympathy and support.

Impact on Dispelling Stereotypes and Fostering Understanding

I strive to be authentic in the curation of my content but am also realistic that our family plays by a different set of rules compared to families led by non-disabled parents. My platforms do afford opportunities to upend stereotypes, but this too must be done with care to avoid the inadvertent perpetuation of negative ideas about dwarfism and disability. When I experience success in my career or personal life, it is never because I 'overcame my disability'. I often spotlight the barriers that remain for people with dwarfism and other disabilities because I do not want people to inaccurately conclude that if I can do something, anyone else could and should. The phrase 'overcoming disability' suggests disability itself, or dwarfism is the primary barrier when in my experience and many others', societal attitudes, discrimination and ableism are the more difficult barriers to overcome.

The Role of Disability Advocacy on Social Media

Leveraging an Audience for Disability Advocacy

My career as a professor frequently offers me the opportunity to speak to audiences about dwarfism and disability. My students represent a wide range of disciplines in healthcare and I am frequently invited to speak to larger audiences or professionals outside the healthcare field. I leverage these engagements to dispel myths and, most importantly, promote the inclusion of people with disabilities. Still, even large speaking engagements pale in comparison to the sizes of audiences reached by a viral social media post. Unlike my 30–90-minute talks, however, I usually have only a few seconds of someone's fleeting attention to make my point in a social media post. The medium can lack context and nuance. Even without much context, social media can spur immediate action. I, and many other advocates, have utilised social media to apply public pressure in an effort to make changes (Andrews et al., 2021). Online dwarfism communities have leveraged social media to gather signatures and calls to stop degrading and dehumanising 'midget wrestling' events (Bulwa, 2023).[3] Events such as these and other stereotypical portrayals of dwarfism are not universally condemned by the community as some prioritise individual choice to participate in these events over the collective harm they bring to the community. The larger disability community is also heterogeneous and sometimes divided in calls for advocacy and action. Some issues, including regulations that would mandate hospitals and clinics to have height-adjustable exam tables (National Council on Disability, 2023), have more universal support than others.

Unpacking Inspiration Porn: Understanding the Phenomenon

In acknowledging the power of social media to prompt change, it is tempting to engage in practices that attract the largest audiences, regardless of their impact on the people they portray. Inspiration porn is extraordinarily viral in its tendency to spread widely across the internet. Despite pushback from disability advocates, social media platforms are still littered with examples of inspiration porn. Stella Young, a person with dwarfism, defined inspiration porn in her renowned 2014 Ted Talk as seemingly commonplace actions (e.g. a child with a visible disability playing with other children) presented as extraordinary or evidence of overcoming disability itself. Young (2014) and others have highlighted the dangers of inspiration porn as dismissing the social barriers that preclude many people with disabilities from full participation in their communities. 'The only disability in life is a bad attitude', is a phrase commonly added to images of disabled people, including little people before it is shared across the internet. By equating disability to a bad attitude, it erases the possibility to positively identify as disabled while also objectifying the individual pictured in the meme. The pictures used for these memes often capture people living their everyday lives and caption the scene as one that should be pitied or celebrated as if entirely unexpected.

I do not want images of me or my family to be characterised in this way but am also aware that many people find themselves to be the subject of this content after pictures were taken without their consent. Inspiration porn perpetuates ableism, or the idea that non-disabled people are superior, because it casts people with disabilities as objects of pity in someone else's story (Grue, 2016). While often wildly popular online, these portrayals disempower and devalue people with disabilities. Evidence in the form of photos or videos of these acts are often taken and shared without the consent of the subject. When people with disabilities push back expressing feelings of exploitation and invasions of privacy, they are often met with claims of ownership over images even of children because they offer a 'feel-good moment' for the non-disabled people who captured and share them.

---

[3]The word 'midget' was used to describe people with dwarfism who were on public display for the curiosity of others. It is a derogatory slur.

Prioritising Quality Over Quantity in Media Representation

To even begin to counter the massive tidal waves of online reach achieved by examples of degrading content, such as inspiration porn, desperation porn (Ayers & Reed, 2022) and other ableist content, it can be argued that we need *more* content that promotes acceptance of dwarfism. We can also offset negative content by amplifying high-quality content that challenges stereotypes while also showcasing the diversity of people with dwarfism.

The Aim: Reduction of Ableist Portrayals Without Censorship

With yet another call for balance, it is important to reduce ableist portrayals of dwarfism in social media while avoiding extensive censorship. There will be varying views on what makes a post or an image authentic. People will have various levels of comfort with how much they share about themselves or their families. It is imperative that we empower people with dwarfism to write and share their own stories – in whatever form they choose. Social media is increasingly accessible to most people, which offers an equitable avenue to reach others with a message or messages of individual choice. We can reclaim the power of telling our own stories and as Uncle Ben famously tells Peter Parker (Spider-Man, Vol. 1, #15, 1962), 'With great power, comes great responsibility'.

Conclusion

This chapter offered my candid insights as a digital content creator with dwarfism who has more than 20 years of experience sharing glimpses from my life as a mother, researcher and community member on social media. It is through a series of intentional acts to share content that is authentic, engaging and resonates with audiences all while maintaining our dignity. While the potential harms of social media, like the sharing of inspiration and desperation porn, are persistent, so too are the innumerable benefits of connection, advocacy and reminding the world, 'We are here'.

References

Andrews, E. E., & Ayers, K. (2016). Parenting with disability: Experiences of disabled women. In S. E. Miles-Cohen & C. Signore (Eds.), *Eliminating inequities for women with disabilities: An agenda for health and wellness* (pp. 209–225). American Psychological Association. https://doi.org/10.1037/14943-011

Andrews, E. E., Ayers, K. B., Brown, K. S., Dunn, D. S., & Pilarski, C. R. (2021). No body is expendable: Medical rationing and disability justice during the COVID-19 pandemic. *American Psychologist*, 76(3), 451–461. https://doi.org/10.1037/amp0000709

Apollo.io. (n.d.). Disaboom.com company information. *Apollo.io* [online]. https://www.apollo.io/companies/Disaboom-com/54a12b0c69702d9ebc424202?chart=count. Accessed on August 07, 2023.

Ayers, K. B., & Reed, K. A. (2022). Inspiration porn and desperation porn: Disrupting the objectification of disability in media. In P. Bones, J. S. Guillion, & D. Barber (Eds.), *Redefining disability* (pp. 90–101). Brill. https://doi.org/10.1163/9789004512702_014

Bacino, C. A. (2023). Achondroplasia. In S. Hahn (Ed.), *UpToDate*. Wolters Kluwer. https://www.uptodate.com/contents/achondroplasia#:~:text=Achondroplasia%20is%20the%20most%20common,receptor%203%20(FGFR3)%20gene. Accessed on October 23, 2023.

Backstrom, L. (2012). From the freak show to the living room: Cultural representations of dwarfism and obesity. *Sociological Forum, 27*(3), 682–707.

Baker, B., & Yang, I. (2018). Social media as social support in pregnancy and the postpartum. *Sexual & Reproductive Healthcare, 17,* 31–34.

Balasubramanian, M. (2023). Osteogenesis imperfecta: An overview. In H. V. Firth (Ed.), *UpToDate*. Wolters Kluwer. https://www.uptodate.com/contents/osteogenesis-imperfecta-an-overview?search=osteogenesis%20imperfecta&source=search_result&selectedTitle=1~70&usage_type=default&display_rank=1. Accessed on October 23, 2023.

Bulwa, D. (2023, July 29). Sonoma county fair wrestling grapples with inclusion. *San Francisco Chronicle* [online]. https://www.sfchronicle.com/bayarea/article/sonoma-county-fair-wrestling-18267987.php. Accessed on November 15, 2023.

Disaboom. (n.d.). Wikipedia [October 2, 2023]. https://en.wikipedia.org/wiki/Disaboom. Accessed on August 07, 2023.

Goffman, E. (1963). *Stigma: Notes on the management of spoiled identity*. Simon and Shuster, Inc.

Grue, J. (2016). The problem with inspiration porn: A tentative definition and a provisional critique. *Disability & Society, 31*(6), 838–849.

Lee, S. (1962). Spiderman. *Amazing Fantasy, 1*(15).

Limoncin, E., Carta, R., Gravina, G. L., Carosa, E., Ciocca, G., Di Sante, S., & andJannini, E. A. (2014). The sexual attraction toward disabilities: A preliminary internet-based study. *International Journal of Impotence Research, 26*(2), 51–54.

Maharlouei, N. (2016). The importance of social support during pregnancy. *Women's Health Bulletin, 3*(1), 1.

National Council on Disability. (2023, May 30). Response to AHRQ request for comments on healthcare delivery of preventive services for people with disabilities. *National Council on Disability*. https://ncd.gov/publications/2023/response-ahrq-request-comments-healthcare-delivery-preventive-services-people. Accessed on September 15, 2023.

Pritchard, E. (2017). Cultural representations of dwarfs and their disabling affects on dwarfs in society. *Considering Disability,* 1–7.

Pritchard, E. (2021). Using Facebook to recruit people with dwarfism: Pros and pitfalls for disabled participants and researchers. *Scandinavian Journal of Disability Research, 23*(1).

Young, S. (2014, April). I'm not your inspiration, thank you very much [Video]. *TEDxSydney*. https://www.ted.com/talks/stella_young_i_m_not_your_inspiration_thank_you_very_much?language=se. Accessed on September 15, 2023.

Chapter 11

Podcasts as a Platform for Advocacy

Jillian Curwin (Writer, Podcast Host, Founder, Owner of Always Looking Up)

USA

Introduction

In 2006, only 22% of adults in the United States were aware of podcasting (Götting, 2023). By 2021 that figure rose to 78%, with researchers estimating that there are an estimated 120 million podcast listeners in the United States (Götting, 2023). Nowadays it seems that there is a podcast for everything, from politics to pop culture, from history to sports and everything in between, ensuring that every listener can find a listening space for them that, in a lot of instances, turns into a community that can encompass the globe. While in this day and age, it seems like everyone has a podcast, they do provide a platform to amplify voices, issues and discord that are not often given attention by the mainstream media.

Like most people I know with dwarfism, I am the only little person in my family (Note, I use little person, dwarf and person with dwarfism interchangeably when talking about myself, all are correct terms). In fact, approximately 80% of people with achondroplasia, the most common type of dwarfism, are born to average-height parents (Foreman et al., 2020). Growing up, I knew that I was different. After all, everyone around me was taller than me, including my younger brother Benjamin. I had sticks screwed into my light switches so that I could reach them, our bathroom sinks were turned sideways and stools were scattered everywhere. What I did not fully comprehend was why I was different, what it meant to be a little person and how those around me actually perceived me, my capabilities and my limitations.

It was not until I was older that I began to comprehend what it truly meant to be a dwarf. It meant living in a world of actual and perceived limits, false beliefs and blatant ignorance, of being objectified and infantilised, of having to constantly combat harmful stereotypes while at the same time trying to justify your humanity. It is also an experience that is quite isolating. As the only dwarf in my world, the only time I was able to see and be a part of the little person community was at the Little People of America (LPA) chapter, regional and national gatherings. At those events, specifically the national conference which takes place annually during a week in the summer, I am able to make eye contact with people, have conversations where no one is talking down to me and be understood by people who simply get my experiences as a dwarf. LPA provides brief moments of normalcy that I feel are often taken for granted by those outside of the community.

I learnt how to advocate for myself through watching my parents advocate for me. Prior to starting kindergarten and elementary school, I watched them in my 504 meetings to explain what accommodations I needed and why.[1] For the most part, they were heard, however, I know of a few accommodations that were made that explicitly were not asked for but the school thought would be best. As I entered middle and high school, the responsibility of not only having to ask for accommodations but making sure those accommodations, were met, fell to me. I had to advocate for myself in order to make sure that I received my second set of textbooks and that I was granted a few extra minutes to get from class to class. However, it is important to note that I did not realise that I was entitled to these accommodations under the Americans with Disabilities Act (1990) and Section 504 of the Rehabilitation Act (1973) because I was disabled. 'Disabled' was not a term I used to identify myself until I was in my mid-20s. I knew to ask for these accommodations because I was a dwarf. Yet, at the same time, I found it frustrating that I had to ask for accommodations that made me stand out when all I wanted at this time in my life was to fit in. So, I pushed back. I said no to certain accommodations that were being made because I saw them as special treatment. I did not want to be special, I wanted to be normal in a world where I knew I could not be. Looking back, I realise that this was a pivotal time where, while I did not, or perhaps could not, grasp what it meant to be a dwarf, to be disabled, I was finding my voice and the skills needed to be heard. Little did I know how those skills would evolve and help define the person, the advocate I would become and the platforms I would build. And it all started with fashion.

In the Beginning – In the Search for Equality

I have had a passion for fashion for as long as I can remember. Vividly I can recall the moment I stumbled across a show called *Project Runway* in the early 2000s and being captivated, the elation at being able to fit into the clothes at Limited Too, then one of the coolest stores for young millennial girls, trying to copy the outfits I saw on the mannequins to the best of my ability. However, I learnt quickly that the fashion industry, like the world around me, is not accessible, it does neither see nor consider little people in the design process and I constantly have to adapt to be on trend. Yet, it is the fashion industry, specifically one moment in fashion history that provided the springboard for me to launch *Always Looking Up*, first the blog and then the podcast. That moment was seeing Sinead

---

[1]Section 504 of the Rehabilitation Act of 1973 (commonly referred to as Section 504) is a federal law designed to protect the rights of individuals with disabilities in programs and activities that receive federal financial assistance.

Burke on the cover of the September 2019 issue of *British Vogue* as one of 15 *Forces for Change* selected by Meghan Markle, the Duchess of Sussex. Holding that magazine in my hands, I carried that issue with me everywhere. I finally felt seen by a frustrating industry that I love, even if it was just a glimpse. It was after my fifth or sixth reread that I realised that I too wanted to be a force for change, that I wanted to use the advocacy skills I had developed over the years out of necessity and survival and start writing about my experiences and perspective on the fashion industry with the hope of changing it for the better.

Always Looking Up, the blog, launched in January 2020. The title comes from the fact that yes, as a little person, I am often looking up at the world around me. For the first three months of the blog, the posts I would write would be from a fashion lens. I would write about what it means to finally own three pairs of jeans that truly fit, describe the process of buying clothes and needing them to be altered, comment on my favourite runway and red carpet looks and hypothesise if they could work for a dwarf body, and advocate for greater dwarfism representation and inclusion in the fashion industry. And then COVID-19.

The fashion industry, like the rest of the world, came to a standstill amidst the onset of the Coronavirus pandemic. Suddenly there were no awards or runway shows to cover, and shopping in-person was not an option. I knew I wanted to continue writing, so I began talking about other issues affecting the dwarfism community such as media representation, or lack thereof, and the lack of accessibility and inclusion across all industries. As luck would have it, a certain film was released in the United States that made a major impact on my life, my identity and my advocacy. That film was *Crip Camp*.

Crip Camp is a documentary film co-directed by Jim LeBrecht and Nicole Newnham and executively produced by the Obamas and the Ford Foundation. *Crip Camp* tells the story of the campers of Camp Jened, a summer camp in upstate New York for teens with disabilities, who would later become leaders of the Disability Rights Movement (Sedgwick, 2021). Activists featured included Judy Heumann, Denise Sherer Jacobson, Brad Lomax and Ed Roberts. It documented the fight for landmark disability rights legislation, specifically the Rehabilitation Act of 1973 and the Americans With Disabilities Act of 1990, highlighting the 504 Sit-Ins.

The 504 Sit-ins of 1977 were in response to the Carter administration's failure to pass regulations regarding the implementation of Section 504, which states that 'no otherwise qualified handicapped individual in the United States shall solely on the basis of his handicap, be excluded from the participation, be denied the benefits of, or be subjected to discrimination under any programme or activity receiving federal financial assistance' (Cone, 2022). To compel the Carter administration to act, disability rights groups in cities across the country occupied federal buildings. Notably, the San Francisco occupation of the Federal Building at 50 United Nations Plaza was one of the largest, a proud display of intersectionality between different civil rights groups and lasted 28 days, to this date the longest occupation of a United States federal building (Crowley, 2024).

The release of the documentary and the conversations I had afterwards with people in the disabled community demonstrated that I had much to learn about my history, my identity and I had a choice to make. I could either continue to live in my ignorance, choose to only focus on dwarfism-specific issues, or I could learn. I could learn what it means to be disabled, how we got to where we are now and how to be an advocate within this incredibly dynamic and diverse community that I did not know but wanted to understand. I chose the latter. I expanded my platform that I was still building, still trying to figure out what I wanted it to be, to talk about issues impacting the disability community.

Are You Listening? Advocating Through Podcasts

Fast forward to May of 2021 when I made the decision to launch my podcast, *Always Looking Up*. I had been floating the idea around in my head for a while but did not know exactly how to do it and if people would listen. But I had been doing this series on my blog called 'Girl Talk' where I would interview my friends in the little person community, the disability community at large, and allies on topics ranging from health and wellness to fashion to accessibility to sports and everything in between, then taking days, sometimes weeks, to transcribe these interviews and publish them on my blog. The process was arduous, and I quickly realised that my guest's voice was getting lost in the transcription. As a result, I reached out to my younger brother Benjamin who, at the time, was a Radio, Television and Film major at Northwestern University, to see if he would be interested in being the podcast's editor and producer. He said yes and the decision was made. *Always Looking Up – The Podcast* was born.

At first, as with 'Girl Talk', my first guests were friends and family, people that I knew I could have an easy and impactful conversation with. Easy was simple. Easy was safe. Prior to each interview, I would write out a list of questions based on where I thought I wanted the conversation to go, and I would ask them as if I were checking items off a list, even if it did not relate to what was said before. The conversations flowed but were certainly, for lack of a better word, choppy. After the first few episodes my brother, who grew up dwarfism-adjacent, familiar with the little person community but not of the little person community, called me out for it. He said to have a list of bullet points but not a list of questions, to let the conversation flow wherever it wants. It did not take long for me to realise how right he was.

The first conversation where I used this new approach was with Rebecca Cokley, who is also a little person. Rebecca is a Programme Officer at the Ford Foundation, the first US Programme Officer to oversee a Disability Rights portfolio. Prior to joining the Foundation in 2021 she was the co-founder and director of the Disability Justice Initiative at the Center for American Progress and served as the executive director for the National Council on Disability. She is also a three-time presidential appointee, serving in the Departments of Education and Health and Human Services under President Barack Obama. She is someone that people look up to in the dwarfism and disability communities, myself included.

On Rebecca's first episode, entitled 'Rebecca Cokley On Being A Disability Rights Activist' we discussed her career up until that point, what it meant to be a disabled advocate in 2021, and the changes she is striving to create in the world. In my conversation with her, listening to her personal story, her words of wisdom, I discovered not only what my podcast could be, but a deeper understanding of the advocate I wanted to be. Rebecca, unlike me, grew up in the advocacy space. She is a second-generation little person, meaning her parents were also little people, from the San Francisco Bay Area and her parents' friends were activists and leaders in the Disability Rights Movement as seen in *Crip Camp*. In our first conversation on the podcast, Rebecca would talk about what milestone events in the disability rights movement she not only saw but played an active role in and it made me realise how young our movement is and that there is no age requirement to being a part of it.

Rebecca, as of this writing, would come on my podcast two more times. The second episode, entitled 'Rebecca Cokley On A Year Of Always Looking Up' was a celebration of a year of the podcast and a discussion on why it is so important to know and preserve dwarfism history and a contemplation of how the definition of being a little person will evolve in the years to come. Her third time was an emergency episode quickly pulled together after the Supreme Court's decision in *Dobbs v. Jackson Women's Health Organization*, was leaked to the public. Their decision overruled *Roe v. Wade* and *Planned Parenthood v. Casey*, which protected the legal right for a woman to have an abortion under the 14th Amendment and returned the power to regulate abortion back to the states. Rebecca and I, along with Bekah Bailey, a little person activist and organiser based in Minneapolis, in the episode entitled 'Bekah Bailey and Rebecca Cokley On How One Decision Impacts The Little Person Community' discussed how we felt in the moment as women, as little people, as disabled people while, at the same time and across the country, it seemed everyone was trying to grapple with the truth of this decision.

Within 24 hours of the news breaking, we were on the microphone recording and had the episode edited and distributed 48 hours later (I should note that this could not have been without an amazing editor and producer working behind the scenes alongside me to make this possible). In the age of the 24-hour news cycle, immediacy is imperative. Particularly at this critical juncture in the women's and disability rights there were a lot of voices ringing out at the same time and it was important to amplify the voices of those speaking up and speaking out in the dwarfism community mainly because, in disability-centred conversations, I have observed that the voices of people with dwarfism are not often heard or even considered. For example, I knew that the Dobbs decision had significant consequences for the dwarfism community and nobody was talking about it, perhaps because nobody knew the impact it would have. It meant that women living in states with strict abortion bans could not get medically necessary treatment should their child be diagnosed with double-dominant dwarfism, a condition that is fatal (Flynn & Pauli, 2003). This episode, perhaps more than any others I have recorded to date, demonstrated the power podcasts have in the advocacy space. They provide a platform for conversations and resources to be shared that are perhaps being ignored, whether accidentally or intentionally, by the mainstream media.

It is not often that you get to speak to people you look up to, people who have empowered you to build your platforms, to follow your dreams, but through the podcast I have the honour of doing just that. Having Rebecca Cokley on the show paved the way for me to speak with other leaders in the disability community such as Maria Town, President and CEO of the American Association of People With Disabilities (AAPD), Emily Voorde, Founder and CEO of INTO Strategies, Haben Girma, notable disability rights attorney and Judy Heumann, international disability rights advocate and regarded as the mother of the disability rights movement. We discussed the many ways they are changing the world through advocacy for people with disabilities through education, litigation, lobbying, drafting policies, etc.

However, it is important to note that the scope of disability advocacy is not limited to the laws and policies. The world, the environment a predominantly non-disabled society has created, is inherently and structurally ableist and there remain many spaces where disability, where dwarfism, is neither seen nor heard. This includes but is not limited to the fashion industry, sports, movies, scripted and reality television, theatre, the more traditional news media, etc. the list is seemingly endless. It is why the conversations I had with Katy Sullivan, Tony nominee, Lucy Jones, Founder and CEO of FFORA, Sami Sage, Founder and CEO of Betches Media and Logan Aldridge, Peloton instructor were equally as important to my advocacy efforts. Representation matters. If disabled people are not seen in certain spaces, then those spaces will not be made accessible.

Conclusion

Podcasts are powerful. Each episode creates a space for ideas for change to be shared and lessons to be learnt. Disability specific organisations such as Little People of America, the OI Foundation, AAPD and numerous others no longer have to wait to be given a platform in order to be heard. All they need is a microphone and the ability to engage in conversation to create a platform for themselves, their community and their cause. People will listen. After all, they are listening now.

References

Cone, K. (2022, March 23). Short history of the 504 sit in. *Disability Rights Education & Defense Fund* [online]. https://dredf.org/504-sit-in-20th-anniversary/short-history-of-the-504-sit-in/. Accessed on January 22, 2024.

Crowley, M. (2024). Disability history: The 1977 504 sit-in. *Disability Rights Florida* [online]. https://disabilityrightsflorida.org/blog/entry/504-sit-in-history. Accessed on January 22, 2024.

Flynn, M. A., & Pauli, R. M. (2003). Double heterozygosity in bone growth disorders: Four new observations and review. *American Journal of Medical Genetics, Part A*, *121A*(3), 193–208. https://doi.org/10.1002/ajmg.a.20143

Foreman, P. K., van Kessel, F., van Hoorn, R., van den Bosch, J., Shediac, R., & Landis, S. (2020). Birth prevalence of achondroplasia: A systematic literature review and meta-analysis. *American Journal of Medical Genetics, Part A*, *182*(10), 2297–2316. https://doi.org/10.1002/ajmg.a.61787

Götting, M. C. (2023). U.S. podcasting industry – Statistics & facts. *Statista* [online]. https://www.statista.com/topics/3170/podcasting/#topicOverview. Accessed on November 22, 2023.

Sedgwick, M. (2021). Review of crip camp co-directed by James LeBrecht and Nicole Newnham. *Disability Studies Quarterly*, *41*(1).

Chapter 12

The Patchwork Representation We Too Often Miss

Sam Drummond (Author)

Australia

May be: The Elephant in the Room?

A reflection on how the journey of working in media and writing a warts and all memoir has challenged the representations of dwarfism in other forms of storytelling.

Everyone has those childhood books that stick with them. The sort that will sit on your shelf all through school and into early adulthood until, if you have children, they are passed onto the next generation as if you planned it all along. But secretly, you just wanted to keep it for yourself. For me, one of those books was *Elmer the Patchwork Elephant*.

'Elmer was different', reads the opening line. 'Elmer was patchwork. Elmer was yellow and orange and red and pink and purple and blue and green and black and white. Elmer was *not* elephant colour' (McKee, 1989, p. 1). Elmer becomes tired of being different from the other elephants. There is a reason Elmer has resonated across the decades for so many people, not least for people with disabilities. From the very start of our lives, we are measured against a medical view of normality and conditioned to shun differences.

When the sonographer scanned me in the womb, my parents breathed a sigh of relief as all the measurements came up as 'normal'. On the day of my birth, my Mum and Dad did not blink an eye as the doctor pronounced my length and weight were in the 'normal' range. But by the time I was 18 months old, my growth had dipped well below average. My family went from doctor to specialist and back again, trying to figure out what was happening. As a man with a stethoscope draped over his off-white collared shirt pronounced that I had pseudoachondroplasia[2] – a form of dwarfism that impacts the size of my limbs and the health of my joints – my parents must have been terrified about what the future held.

I was different. This was not part of the plan. They had spent their whole lives being told what an ideal human looked like, and I was not it. I had a disability.

And it would impact the way I experienced the world around me, and how the world around me would experience me. Most of these experiences have been moulded by representations in books, films and mainstream media.

Growing up, I had no problem finding representations of myself. What I did see was the overrepresentation of one-dimensional characters. These were people on the sidelines, without power and without a voice. I was one of Snow White's dwarfs, defined by a single emotion. I was an Oompa Loompa, ripe for exploitation by an eccentric billionaire. I was a hyper-sexualised Mini-Me, a voiceless object of ridicule.

Not only did these representations shape the views I had of myself, they also shaped the views that others had of me and what they thought I was capable of. Growing up in a small town, I would often make an appearance in the local paper. But it was too often a story of limitations – a sports star bending down to be at my level in the photo or an award for excellence in being disabled. There was a distinct lack of agency. It was charity through media.

When I moved from the country to the city to pursue my studies – away from the safety provided by Mum – I discovered these representations of disability and dwarfism flowed through the suburbs like a cancer through the bloodstream. People at bars and clubs ridiculed me or made sexualised jokes. Drivers yelled abuse out their car windows. Potential employer ignored me. This is the reality for so many people with dwarfism. We are talked about, written about and portrayed, but too rarely are we given a pen or a microphone. All of this has been the subject of my recent memoir *Broke* (see, Drummond, 2023).

Broke

The story involves a broken family. It involves the process of breaking my bones to straighten them, in an attempt to fit my body to what the medical textbooks said people should look like. It involves rural disadvantage, insecure work, a social safety net that only works in some cases. Spoiler alert – there are no convenient plot twists, no inspirational moment of realisation and no happy ending. Real life is not so kind to storytellers. It would not have been honest of me to wrap things up with a nice little bow on top. Nevertheless, people often ask me what comes next. My bio says I am a media maker, a human rights lawyer, an author, a partner and a father. All of these titles seemed pretty unlikely for the disabled kid from the country who was struggling to find his place in the wider world. What happened after the final scenes of the book that allowed that to happen?

One of the answers lies in the protagonist of *Broke* – my Mum. She sacrificed much, including her own health, for the slim chance that my brother and I would be able to follow our dreams. I was down and out. I could not find secure housing, had no money, my health was suffering and I had not found *my people*. Folks were giving me all sorts of advice on what I should do. People told me I should get a job, but that was easier said than done. Potential employers sounded keen over the phone, but their reactions changed once they saw me, asking things like 'how will you reach the top shelf?' or just saying 'we'll call you'. They never did. Once again, I was defined by the representations we had all been fed about people like me.

It certainly never occurred to me that I could have my own voice. That is until I started listening to my local community radio station. The invitation was made on air for people to do the radio training course, and I signed up. I did the course. I got a show. It was about cheese. I did more shows – about blues music, about sport, a radio show about television shows. About my favourite musician, Jack White. About sex and relationships, much to my Dad's dismay.

These were all things that I wanted to talk about. It was revolutionary. I had found my people, this bunch of misfits who found solace in a rundown studio. Most importantly, I had found my voice. It led me to working alongside some of the most experienced media makers in Australia. It led to a workplace where every day without fail, I would hear the wheels of a powered chair coming up behind me and a voice telling people who already had a national platform that they wanted to talk to me and not them. The wheels belonged to disability activist, Stella Young who was working down the corridor.

We had both connected years earlier through community media. She was hosting her community TV show *No Limits* when I was behind a microphone at the radio station down the street. By the time we were in the same building, she was editing the ABC's dedicated space for disabled voices *Ramp Up* and had just recorded her groundbreaking TED talk in which she declared 'I am not your inspiration'.

'What are you going to write for me this week?' she would ask when she came to my desk.

Suddenly, my perspective was unique, and it was powerful. My voice was being heard. But still it felt like some secret society of disabled media makers pushing our message after being told our whole lives there was something wrong with us – when it was, in fact, society that had the problem.

We whispered words of encouragement to each other. How are we going to tell our stories to get this message out there? I had been struggling to get any sort of work at all. Now the opportunities started flooding in. I got great jobs, made lifelong friends, won awards, met my life partner and became a father. That's how a bio happens, it seems. Even then, the challenge was never over.

Stella and I were asked to be part of a book about people with dwarfism by someone without dwarfism. We were both interviewed for the book as another opportunity to get our perspectives out there. When the book landed on my desk and I started reading, my jaw dropped. This first-person account claiming to me was not my words. I had been misquoted. My experiences had been altered. My ideas had been bastardised. I picked up the phone to Stella. She was mid-sentence when she answered.

'Are you reading this shit?' she asked.

Once again, someone with the best of intentions was stealing our voice and cheapening our stories. We were left powerless. This book now sits on my shelf next to *Broke* as a reminder of the need to let disabled people tell their own stories, not pretending to speak on their behalf. All this led to a realisation that I had been hiding all this time.

For those who have not grown up on this island continent, not all Australian accents are the same. Mine has a metro base with a hint of country, albeit from the south where we do not have the distinctive Crocodile Dundee twang.[1] My voice is deep and rather loud, unlike many representations of dwarfism in popular culture – think the high pitched squeaks from Snow Whites' dwarfs or the almost complete voicelessness of Mini-Me. My voice is male. My voice is middle Australia.

Radio allowed me to pass myself off as something I was not – non-disabled. An unquestioned member of the privileged majority. The assumptions that people made about me disappeared on the wireless, but in doing so, I lost part of who I was. I was Elmer the elephant, painting himself grey to fit in with everyone else. Back to our elephant hero, Elmer sidles up to the rest of the elephants and realises that that perspective he brought, that spark that made him valuable to the herd, was all but lost.

> Finally he could bear it no longer. He lifted his trunk and at the top of his voice shouted: Booo! (McKee, 1989)

This is what I have felt like in the years since I realised I was hiding behind the microphone. I have done my best to show my true colours, whether it is saying yes to a television interview, standing before an audience on stage or simply getting up on the dance floor. I remember the first time I saw myself on TV. I recoiled in the same way some people do when they hear their own voice. I had got through life pretending that I was like everybody else. I formed close friendships and stuck with them because I knew they would treat me like other people, laughing at my jokes or calling me out when I had done something silly.

I hated meeting strangers or walking down busy streets because of other people's reactions. It was the most obvious time that I could see the prejudice in other people's eyes. In this new world of seeing myself from the camera's perspective, I tried to embrace the discomfort. If I am being challenged by seeing myself, I thought, then others are too. This is representation.

As a society, we have become terrible at understanding each other's positions. We lock ourselves in our bubbles and refuse – deliberately or not – to see the other side of the story. It is impossible to understand each other until we have walked in each other's shoes. Or in my case, waddled in my shoes, wheeled in a wheelchair, jumped along on crutches. That is why I decided to write a book. I have had the honour of being part of a number of books – chapters as part of a broader story, but this would be my story. My family's story. A message to people in power that they need to shift their focus. A signal to people in similar situations that they are not alone.

---

[1] *Crocodile Dundee* is a 1986 action comedy film. The protagonist is crocodile hunter Mick Dundee (Paul Hogan) has what is referred to as a broad Australian accent.

Then came the next step. Writing it all down. It took writing every night for a year, after the bedtime of a talkative two-year-old. At the end of each chapter, I would collapse with the emotional load of it all. But once I started writing, I had to finish. The result is *Broke*, a memoir about growing up with a disability in a single parent family in Australia and the highs and lows that come with that. It is a book that sets out not to tell readers what to think, instead showing them how it tasted, smelt and felt like to be in that situation. My goal was a real representation of disability, warts and all. It is not pretending that everything was terrible or that everything was great? My intention was to show a disabled person as flawed, not because of my disability but because I am human. This is a representation of disability, and indeed dwarfism, that I never saw on my TV screen or in books growing up. I never saw a person with dwarfism as multidimensional. I never realised that being patchwork was a wonderful part of being alive.

Growing up, I could never distinguish between what was disadvantage created by disability or disadvantage for other reasons – living rurally, being in a single parent family, using public health and public education, etc. Writing the book I struggled to think of what people would think was an out-of-the-ordinary life event or what was just an everyday occurrence for people growing up. So I just wrote to just show people what it was like to be me.

Broke deliberately refrains from ramming agendas down readers' throats. There are no references to university studies or policy papers or expert solutions. It is the raw manuscript of what life was like growing up in a single parent family with a disability and everything that entails – insecure housing, reliance on welfare and casual work, well-intentioned people not really helping, bad-intentioned people making things even worse. It seeks to show readers how it tasted, smelt and felt like to be in that situation. Like the feeling of waking up with legs in full plaster and doctors not believing a child that the plaster is too tight until their feet started to turn purple. Or what goes through someone's head when their last option for employment seems to be dressing up as a jockey for drunken revellers. Or even just the taste of junk food as a single mother watches on having a glass of cheap wine as a replacement for dinner.

As a result, I now see the book as a mirror for readers' own lives. People's reactions are invariably to the bits in which they saw themselves. This has included being a single parent, growing up in the 1990s, attending government schools or even something as specific as the coins people throw in shopping centre fountains. My hope is that people with disabilities, in particular people with dwarfism, can identify themselves and find solace that they are not alone.

At the end of Elmer, it starts to rain.

> When the rain fell on Elmer, his patchwork started to show again.
> (McKee, 1989, p. 5)

Broke is just another way that I try to make sure my patchwork is showing. This is a constant process. The way the media shaped my views of myself will be with me forever. But by constantly revealing myself, I say to the world – 'this is me, I'm disabled and I'm proud'. Perhaps one day, people with disabilities will not have to explain themselves to fit in at all. Perhaps one day, we will be truly accepted and embraced for the unique perspective we bring to the human story.

References

Drummond, S. (2023). *Broke*. Affirm Press.
McKee, D. (1989). *Elmer the patchwork elephant* (2nd ed.). Andersen Press.

Chapter 13

'Would You Befriend Me, Date Me, Hire Me if I Hadn't Had My Bones Broken & Stretched to Look More Like Yours?'

Emily Sullivan Sanford (Freelance Author)

Germany

'Was it *really* your choice to do it if you were that young when you started it?' That's the question I hear the most when someone learns I underwent limb-lengthening procedures from ages 11 to 17 that lengthened my shins, upper arms and thigh bones. The result gained me a foot (30 cm) of height and longer arms that are more proportional to my body.

It would be a lie to deny that my parents were fully on board. But it would also be a lie to omit that they ensured I felt the choice was mine. That feeling was essential. It validated the fact that even if the non-dwarf adults in my life simply wanted the best for me, only I knew how it felt to have dwarfism. Only I knew how it felt to face the chance to alter one's body so drastically through such dramatic measures. And I knew, to the core of my being, that I was never, ever motivated to do it because I was ashamed to have dwarfism.

I chose limb-lengthening to access public facilities – desks, shelves, counters, cash registers, ATMs, clothing racks, hotel shower heads, exercise equipment, rental cars and rental bikes – without any modifications. I did it to use public seats – classroom chairs, restaurant chairs, theatre seats, train seats, plane seats, toilets, friends' furniture – without needing footstools to keep my legs from dangling and falling asleep. I did it to correct some of my lordosis so that I would no longer need to carry backrests with me to every desk chair I sat in.[1] I did it to have the extra leverage enabling me to lug more around: bigger suitcases, bigger shopping bags, bigger backpacks, bigger children. I did it to take bigger steps when walking, so I could cover more ground before I got tired. I did it to stop straining to reach the back of my head when brushing my hair. Looking back on it all now, almost 25 years since I finished the last procedure, this reason was enough for me.

---

[1] A severe curvature of the lower spine caused by achondroplastic dwarfism.

But my limb-lengthening has inspired others to react differently to me and my body than if I had grown up to look like a typical person with achondroplasia. Many non-dwarfs assume something is up when they see me. Most questions from kids are about my gait. Adults usually ask about my scars in the warm months when I wear short sleeves and dresses. My husband saw them and assumed I had been in a car accident the night we first met. Someone else was brazen enough to ask me this outright during a job interview, much to my astonishment. A few times, I've been told a story of two acquaintances talking about my diagnosis behind my back, summed up to me thusly: 'They were like, "I couldn't even tell she was a dwarf!" and I was like, "What are you, nuts? It's so obvious!"'

Such speculation aside, the social benefits of limb-lengthening are undisputable. I have never been photographed on the street. Strangers never shout, mutter or whisper slurs associated with dwarfism at me. They don't try to pick me up. No one asks where my parents are, mistaking me for a child. The risks of being confronted with such reactions are high for people with visible markers of dwarfism pretty much every single time they go out in public. I no longer face such risks. In fact, on several occasions, I've heard acquaintances and co-workers use ableist slurs to denigrate someone else in my presence, as in, 'That guy looked all hunched over and pathetic like some little midget!'[2]

Revealing my medical history is an act of trust, one that some have betrayed. A friend of a friend referred to me as 'Dwarf Emily' but only behind my back. Another made lewd comments fetishising my body and my dwarfism after a date. I have never attempted to conceal my diagnosis to someone to spare me such hurt. I sometimes decide against disclosure simply because it doesn't seem relevant, or I've merely forgotten to. But experience has taught me that the degree to which I'll be perceived as physically 'normal' is something I ultimately cannot control. My best bet is to be open and own my story as much as I can.

That sense of ownership was crucial for the years I spent limb-lengthening because the second most frequent question I hear about my surgeries is, 'Would you do it again?' I can't answer this without more specifics. If you mean, would I do it knowing now exactly how painful, how long, how intense it would be? Probably. If you mean, would I be willing to go through it all twice? Unlikely. It was more painful than you can imagine, and there were risks.

First, there is the chronic pain you endure every single day of the months-long lengthening process: the aching from the muscles and bones being stretched, from the exercises in physical therapy meant to combat the stiffening of the muscles and the sting of having salt literally rubbed into the open wounds to sterilise them. Heavy painkillers are prescribed with side effects that do a number on your appetite and sometimes your sleep. On top of these daily pains, sudden severe pain crops up frequently. There are burning infections at the pin sites that flare up from you having touched your wounds with unsterilised hands. (Every kid does this, despite warnings not to, just as every kid scratches itchy mosquito bites.)

---

[2]Derived from the word 'midge', this term has been considered offensive in dwarf communities for roughly 50 years. Non-dwarf speakers use the term today out of either malice or ignorance.

There is acute pain that reverberates deep in your bones when you accidentally bang a metal fixator against something hard or ride in a car that drives over a pothole. And then there are the scenes worthy of cinema, like when I got a searing muscle cramp deep in my thigh after a fixator had been adjusted, which left me screaming as hard as I could for a good 15 minutes and then whimpering for another two hours. Or when another fixator on my arm had somehow managed to jump the track and had to be forced back into place. Or when pins were unscrewed from my thigh bone and the pain matched the fact that the femur is the biggest bone in the body. Or the panic attacks, dry heaving and hallucinations I developed from certain analgesics. Or the infection that wouldn't go away because I had developed a resistance to antibiotics after so many infections. Or the fever, chills, vomiting and insomnia that lasted a full week, which my doctors suspected resulted from my having undergone three major surgeries in 6 months. This is what some dwarfs endure to protect themselves from ableism.

It starts to sound like we endured torture, and there are plenty of critics who characterise limb-lengthening as such. Did it make me stronger, or did it instil lasting trauma? Both. In terms of strength gained, having dwarfism and undergoing limb-lengthening have been among the most important adventures of my life because I have never doubted what they mean to me. Feeling that limb-lengthening was my choice is what kept me going when the pain was so bad that my mother asked if I wanted to stop the process then and there. I may not have been quite this eloquent in the moment, but my reply went something like this: '*I* got myself into this. *I'm* seeing it to the end because I'm doing it for myself. This is my pain that I have to face to keep going. I know I can do it'. The night before beginning any one of the procedures, I insisted on sitting next to my parents as the list of surgical risks was read out before they signed the waiver. I wanted to know exactly what I was getting into. I chose not to have my scars cosmetically removed as a reminder to myself of what I achieved and why I did it.

The procedures also left me in some ways traumatised. To this day, I startle easily and often overreact with a loud gasp, a relic of my having experienced muscle spasms whenever I was bumped or heard a sudden sound during the lengthening period. My years in hospitals have rendered me unable to fall asleep in such places without medication, something I learned as an adult when I spent five straight nights wide awake and rather delirious. Worst of all, my anterior tibialis tendons on both of my ankles were accidentally severed at some point during my first limb-lengthening, which now makes me stumble about every few weeks and makes dismounting from a bicycle dangerous. After two surgeries to repair the tendons and three years of physical therapy, they remain weak. One non-dwarf parent opposed to most elective surgeries for disabled minors told me point-blank, 'Well, that's what you got for having limb-lengthening'.

I was sorry to hear this was their primary take on my story because the greatest impact on my life from limb-lengthening came not from any physical trauma *or* triumph but from the great shift in perspective that came from using a wheelchair and living in a paediatric rehabilitation centre for several months. Until limb-lengthening, I had spent my life as the most physically remarkable child in almost any setting, save for annual doctor's check-ups and Little People of

America meetings. With fixators on both legs and living in an institution, I suddenly found myself more disabled than I had ever been and friends with kids who were more severely and permanently disabled than I ever would be.

My parents and brother can easily attest to the frustration, fury and melancholy I often vented during limb-lengthening, but my mood shifted abruptly each week when I attended adolescent group therapy, where my condition and treatment rendered me the most privileged in the room. I had dwarfism, of which I was proud. I was undergoing limb-lengthening, which would make me taller. I wasn't on a waiting list for a round-the-clock caregiving service because my family refused to have me at home. I had never been told by a parent or *any* of my relatives, 'I wish you'd never been born'. I often left group therapy shaken. 'How can her mom not want her at home?!' I asked my own mom. It was so hard to believe, but the experience ultimately forced me to believe such things, and that made the wrongs inflicted by systemic ableism all the easier for me to believe as I grew up. I would never trade these humbling experiences for a more normal adolescence, whatever that is supposed to be.

They compelled me to see things from other points of view, which also helped me navigate the heated debates surrounding limb-lengthening itself. I was aware of the controversy early on. Although I never lost any of my close friends, most of the dwarf community all but shunned us after my first procedure, while non-dwarf adults generally dismissed the dwarf community as selfish. My parents admitted to me that my own orthopaedist, Dr Steven Kopits – who did not have dwarfism – viewed the procedures as *not worth the pain*. He had spent his life advocating for the empowerment of people with dwarfism, etching himself into the memories of countless parents who said he was that one doctor who urged them to simply love and support their dwarf children. He was often the first to ever call their children 'beautiful' (Adelson, 2005).

This helped me understand that many opposed to the procedures did so in good faith. I had less understanding for the person with dwarfism who approached one of my fellow patients and his mother in a train station and accused his mother of 'ruining' her child's life. She turned to her son after the confrontation and asked him what he thought of it.

'I think you shouldn't speak to strangers', he replied.

Some arguments in favour of limb-lengthening from the non-dwarf people in my life could strike me as equally unhelpful. 'So *what* if you do it to blend in?' a few said to me in an effort to show support. Such comments reminded me that I was still a dwarf, not just because of my fibroblast growth receptor gene but because of the reply that was instantly ready at the tip of my tongue: So *what* if I did it to blend in? Well, it says something pretty miserable about how we treat people who don't blend in if I were convinced I had to undergo a total of 4 years of breaking, stretching and healing six of the biggest bones in my body to avoid that fate, doesn't it?

Anyone who knew my parents well could conclude that their decision to recommend limb-lengthening to me was not one bit motivated by a desire to see me blend in physically. After all, when it came to raising me to be proud of who I was, they did not miss a beat. I knew the word 'dwarf' and felt positively about it before I understood it thanks to their affectionate tone. When I asked about my large skull, I was told, 'Because you have room for an extra package of brains'. When I got swooped up in the hot-pink 1980s storm of Disney princesses and Barbie dolls, my parents regularly tossed out commentary to counteract the dangers of the beauty standard: 'If Barbie were a real woman, she'd be taller than a house and fall over!' 'We gotta tell that Walt Disney that not all dwarfs are bearded men with silly names!' 'I hope the prince doesn't just love Cinderella for her looks because she's not always going to look that way!'

My parents joined the local chapter of Little People of America, where they were suddenly made to feel what it's like to be in the minority as they towered over other members and learned everything there was on offer. Our house was a library of every resource on dwarfism on the market. They travelled great distances, past nearby New York – where the experts on dwarfism had less than stellar reputations – to Baltimore, where the Little People's Research Fund was known to be among the best. But I cannot honestly claim that their reasons for offering to support me through limb-lengthening were purely medical.

A core value in liberal democracies is that medical choices should be made freely. But the parents of any child with a condition that society struggles to accept are not making the choice freely. Whether they are facing the decision to pursue limb-lengthening on a dwarf child, or to continue a pregnancy that tested positive prenatally for Down Syndrome or to adopt a child with any number of severe disabilities, no parent can make such decisions based solely on their own personal skills and circumstances. They face these decisions under enormous pressure from the world, which regularly shows them how cruel it can be to children and adults who don't fit mainstream definitions of beauty and success.

Intersectionality reveals how this cruelty takes different forms depending upon your gender, sexuality and economic background. Ribbing a guy for being short has long been widely accepted, but little attention is paid to the appalling results of this when it escalates. Activist Bill Klein, who has spondyloepiphyseal dysplasia congenita, wrote in his 2015 memoir about harassment at university that drove him to severe depression and suicidal ideation (Arnold & Klein, 2015). The following year, *The Hollywood Reporter* ran an excellent, horrifying exposé on the exploitation of people with dwarfism in the entertainment industry and the resulting mental health crises commonly experienced by the performers, quoting actor Verne Troyer of Mini-Me fame, among others (Abramovitch, 2016). Two years later, Troyer died by suicide. The year before his death, disability rights activist Rebecca Cokely (2017), who has achondroplasia, published 'Little People, Big Depression', writing:

> I think the first time I was made aware of the propensity of Little People to kill themselves was when my mom lost her first love in 1989... I remember my mom's reaction to P's death... I remember her telling me that this is also something that was far too common in the dwarfism community and something that we honestly didn't talk about enough. She hoped that I would never have to go through what she was going through, watching friend after

friend die. It was less than a year later when actor David Rappaport killed himself and I lost my first hero... Since David's death many more little people, actors and non-actors, have committed suicide. I've lost countless more friends than 10-year-old Rebecca the fangirl could've ever guessed (including the first person I seriously dated in the LP community). Both men and women, but many more men.

Across the vast majority of countries, men have higher rates of suicide than women, largely driven by the social expectation that men should be successful and self-reliant in both body and mind. As sociologist Stephanie Coontz (2000) points out, the scorn heaped on a man who sometimes needs support sets off a vicious cycle that will heap further scorn upon him should he seek support.

Even when parents raise their dwarf child to be loved and proud of who they are, no one yet expects them to have opportunities equal to non-dwarfs. The 2001 documentary *Dwarfs: Not A Fairy Tale*, which I appeared in, features Dr Michael Ain, a man with achondroplasia who became a surgeon. A cousin watching the film assumed at first sight that Dr Ain was an orderly. A close friend assumed he was a maintenance worker. One of my in-laws let out a jubilant, 'WOW!' when his true profession was revealed. Hearing their surprise secretly jarred me. Growing up with dwarfism in a caring community, you often hear, 'You can be *anything* you want to be'. Then in young adulthood, you learn there was an unspoken second clause: 'But we'll be genuinely surprised if it works out. Overjoyed for you, absolutely. But quite surprised'.

As I came of age, I found these low expectations weren't off the mark. How often do we see visibly disabled doctors or surgeons? In all my hundreds of medical examinations, I have been treated only once by specialist with a visible disability. I almost hugged him. I was projecting a lot onto him of course, but I felt he *had* to know what it was like to not just look through the microscope but also to be placed under it by doctors whose condescension often shines through.

I had once attended a bioethics conference where an orthopaedic surgeon who had worked for years on dwarfism presented a slide asserting that the abundance of skin and muscle on short limbs makes people with achondroplasia 'look like the Michelin Man'. He smiled, genuinely proud of what he felt was a wry comparison. That years of working with dwarf patients did not inspire him to consider his joke from our perspective spoke volumes to me about the medical establishment. Dr Michael Ain spoke in *Dwarfs* of the macho culture of this establishment, which spurned his eligibility for medical school on the basis of his size.

While reductive definitions of strength and success continue to be the harsh measure of a man, women and other gender minorities are more likely to be assessed by reductive definitions of beauty. Whenever I ask the adult participants in my diversity workshops to name a visibly disabled actress, awkward silence follows every time. The same goes for naming a visibly disabled heroine of a great romance story. *Beauty and the Beast*, *Cyrano De Bergerac* and *The Phantom of the Opera* attest that heroines can look past a man's extraordinary appearance and love them back. But we've yet to see a beloved heroine unveil a severe deformity and hear her strapping lover say, 'I think it's intriguing. And I wanna knock boots with you. So. Bad'. And while disabled women are regularly excluded from the realm of mainstream beauty and romance, disabled people of all genders are covertly fetishised and victimised. The US Justice Department revealed in a 2020 report that disabled people are more than six times more likely to be sexually assaulted than the general population (Harrell, 2021).

People who refuse to try to live up to traditional gender roles too often struggle to find support in more progressive spaces if they are disabled. Girl power voices in the mainstream media that promote self-defence and empowerment through sports repeatedly forget options or imagery that include disabled bodies. The response to the statistics on sexual assault against disabled people pales in comparison to the volume of think-pieces that have ensued when a (non-disabled) celebrity has been accused of assaulting (non-disabled) victims. Through recent films like *Fire Island* and exhibits like 'Cripping the Queer, Queering the Crip' here in Berlin, members of the gay community are just starting to call out its own history of lookism and ableism. Drag performer Damian Fatale, who has Schmid metaphyseal chondrodysplasia, told *Vice* magazine, 'When I was in high school, I would get bullied by the Gay-Straight Alliance members. They would constantly be on me, trying to make sure that I fit impossible standards because they thought I embarrassed all the gay kids at that school. I think it was because I was obviously different and they wanted to be seen as regular people' (Chester, 2015).

It can be deeply upsetting to see callousness towards visibly disabled people persist in circles where equality and diversity are touted as values. The 4 years I attended Bard College – whose student body and staff were consistently ranked among the farthest left in the United States – were 4 years where I heard more snickering about dwarfism than anywhere else. Dwarf-tossing jokes were printed in the student newspaper. The surrealist film club ran a 'dwarf-themed' evening, featuring *The Tin Drum* and *Even Dwarfs Started Off Small* 'because it's just so cool to see the dwarfs go so crazy and ape-shit', according to the promoter. This fixation on objectifying freaks was echoed on our favourite TV show of the time, *Scrubs*, where racism and sexism were frequently called out, but dwarfism was only ever mentioned as a gut-splitting joke.

This is not to say ableism is more widespread than any other prejudice or that people with dwarfism are pushed farther to the margins than any other minority. Those who try to play Oppression Olympics – whether arguing ableism is worse than racism, or cis women have it worse than trans women or Black people are more persecuted than Jewish people – might as well carry around a sign reading, 'I'VE BEEN DIVIDED AND CONQUERED'. It's counterproductive and morally corrupt, signifying a refusal to practise the proactive empathy we demand from others.

The fight against ableism fails without radical empathy. Without it, we are doomed to ignore intersectional injustices and concern ourselves only with those we deem our own kind. Years ago, a woman from the United States belonging to an ethnic minority reached out to me to discuss her daughter's achondroplasia, which her immigrant family dismissed as imaginary, something made up by American doctors that she would surely outgrow. A friend of mine from the same country told me people with disabilities there have few opportunities for self-actualisation, which was likely why the child's loving relatives were in deep denial. Indeed, the dwarf experience varies greatly depending on where you live. The Nordic countries are currently rated among the fairest for people with disabilities. However, the recent rise of populist political parties that scapegoat immigrants and ethnic minorities in the region indicates many of their disabled residents have fewer opportunities and face more discrimination than others.

This is a problem everywhere of course. Across the West, almost all disability advocacy groups have started off overwhelmingly middle class, heteronormative and white, which is not representative of the population. The majority of workers in the United Kingdom and the United States are working class or poor, which means the majority of workers with dwarfism are, too. Racial minorities are on track to become the majority of the US population in the next two decades, ensuring your average American – and your average American dwarfism – will be neither middle class nor white.

For too long, dwarf advocacy has had little to say about the ways in which ableism combines with other chauvinisms. All children with dwarfism begin life faced with the challenge of finding adequate healthcare and the experts to administer it. Recent studies have found racial disparities in referrals to appropriate care, rendering Black children with dwarfism in the United States and the United Kingdom more disadvantaged than white (Davies et al., 2023). We need far more research and resources on such problems in the healthcare sector and beyond. Those of us who teach diversity workshops about dwarfism are hard-pressed to find materials that represent people of colour with dwarfism and that address the specific bigotries they face.

The same goes for people with dwarfism born farther down the class ladder. In any nation with high income inequality and austere social support systems, low-income families are likely to receive a lower quality of care for their dwarf children. Precarious employment leaves such families with few means to travel to the conferences and clinics that specialise in rare conditions or to take time off from work for major medical procedures. Such problems deserve far more attention than they have traditionally been given. Efforts to increase educational and job opportunities for applicants with dwarfism too often concentrate on nondiscrimination policies and accessibility regulations in middle-class workplaces and at universities, forgetting that most dwarfs are not middle class and therefore face more obstacles to such places. Advocating for robust social welfare programmes, universal healthcare, investment in the public schools of every neighbourhood, a living wage, paid leave for workers of all income levels, and far-reaching anti-racist reforms are the responsibilities of anyone committed to disability rights for all disabled people.

It's nice to think any vulnerability to bigotry automatically fuels a willingness to step out of your comfort zone and feel compassion for anyone living on the margins. But we all have blind spots and biases to work through. Damian Fatale found the dwarf community in the United States to be as homophobic as mainstream American culture. Sexologist Dr Marylou Naccarato, who opened the first information booth on sexual satisfaction at a Little People of America convention, attested that such organisations have long maintained oppressively narrow models of love and sexuality, stemming from their roots in family organisations that skew conservative (Gerson, 2014). In the books, documentaries and articles I was raised on, many dwarfs cited these conventions as the place where they sought dates and found love. That queer dwarfs were not welcome to do the same is an injustice that warrants reckoning in the larger dwarf community.

For too many humans, belonging to more than one minority group has historically meant being welcome in neither community, let alone mainstream society. Such ultra-marginalisation has inspired some to seek out fellow outcasts and form their own communities. They deserve unwavering support from both minority rights groups and the mainstream that is long overdue.

Recognising and accommodating the vast diversity that exists within every minority is the only way we can demand justice with a straight face. If we want tolerance from non-disabled people, we must practise it ourselves, and tolerance means figuring out what you're afraid of and why. Limb-lengthening gave me insight into the many ways there are to have a body and the many different reactions such bodies endure. The conversations have shown me that most of us tend to be biased towards medical procedures that make others more like us and biased against procedures that make them more different.

In the current debates on hormone treatments for transgender children, I've heard many voice their opposition because they believe all major body alteration should wait until adulthood.

To this assertion, I always reply, 'It's a valid worry, but are you also opposed to limb-lengthening, which is best done before adulthood when muscles and joints start to stiffen?'

The answer is usually: 'That's different. You *needed* limb-lengthening to function'. Rarely is the speaker more informed about gender dysphoria or achondroplasia than any other random person pulled off the street. The ease with which they imagine one procedure as automatically healing and the other as dangerously regrettable reflects deeply ingrained assumptions of what a person needs to 'function'.

An essential step towards true freedom of choice for patients and parents of underage patients requires an inclusive approach to reporting and debating life-altering medical decisions that recognises the full complexity and range of experience. Organisations, activists and the reporters who spread their message must listen to anyone glad to have undergone limb-lengthening, to anyone who regrets it and to those whose feelings land somewhere in the middle. Silencing or dismissing either side because their experience is less frequent than the other is to contradict the very basis of minority rights.

My story – the whole, complex story – should help to inform others. I denounce reports that elide limb-lengthening into a miraculous cure-all for those 'suffering' from dwarfism, which doctors are seeking to 'combat'. I cringe and sigh when 'before' and 'after' shots of patients feature sweatpants, unwashed hair and grainy resolution in the first photo, and sleek evening wear, makeup and perfect lighting in the second. Conversely, I also speak out when bloggers blithely opine that I must have been 'forced' into having limb-lengthening by parents driven by their need for a child who looked normal.

Everyone should know that limb-lengthening did improve my physical functioning, and that it also cost me abilities I once had. I wish – very often – that my tendons had never been injured by limb-lengthening. I miss cycling and jumping rope. Along with the pain, it was indeed the price I paid for undergoing the procedures. Although I was the first of my surgeon's patients to incur such an injury, this fact is cold comfort to me as I am the one who must live with the consequences. Frustration is frequent but never escalates to regret because exchange is impossible, and risks have accompanied every surgery I have had.

Indeed, everyone should know that having achondroplasia has also been at times difficult and painful for me. Less permanent but more harrowing than my tendon injury from limb-lengthening was an error during a laminectomy procedure I had at age 30 to relieve spinal compression and restore my ability to walk. The surface of my spinal cord was accidentally cut open, resulting in a few days of physical trauma and a fair amount of anxiety until it healed. As of this writing, I have 16 surgeries under my belt, half of which were limb-lengthening. The other half were treatments for secondary conditions resulting from achondroplasia: bowed legs, sleep apnoea, chronic ear infections, uterine fibroids (Allanson & Hall, 1986) and spinal complications. None of these procedures were easy, and most of them were more painful than anyone told me they would be.

The benefits and risks of any major medical procedure are abundant. This is why I could no sooner decide for an individual whether they should undergo limb-lengthening than I could decide whether, when, or how they should have a child. When sharing my experiences, I must beware of the risk of placing pressure on others. Every single one of us who has ever opted for or against a life-changing procedure feels compelled to defend that decision, whatever it was. But anyone who presents their experience as proof of why everyone should make the same decision they did is betraying a self-centeredness that should cost them their credibility.

Patients and parents of underage patients deserve to learn that many procedures considered medically necessary in one place are considered at best elective and at worst damaging in another. They deserve to understand the differences between the social model of disability and the medical model. Such an understanding – fundamental to disability rights – requires we examine our cultural values as much as our bodies until we no longer mistake harmless physical features that may be unfashionable for harmful conditions that must be treated. American kids of my generation were told orthodontic braces were necessary to avoid painful disfiguration. But the cosmetic nature of the procedure comes into question when we consider the ubiquity of bare-teethed smiling in Hollywood, in contrast to other nations, where braces are rare, and it's considered proper etiquette to cover your mouth when you smile broadly enough to show your teeth. From male circumcision to female genital cutting, one culture winces while another shrugs.

As of this writing, bans on gender-affirming care for children have exploded across the United States and other countries as a backlash to the growing transgender rights movement. Although they are said to protect children from procedures they are too young to understand, none of these bans have included restrictions on 'normalising' intersex surgeries for minors or cosmetic breast implants for underage cisgender girls. To reveal your stance on countless issues of bioethics is to reveal your politics and your blind spots.

We must address these blind spots head-on because they create the social pressure that hinders true freedom of choice. No parent wants to see their child hurt or harmed by others. No one wants to imagine their child ever called a freak on the playground, on the street, at a frat party, in bed. No one wants to imagine potential employers choosing their words very carefully to formulate a rejection letter that eludes lawsuits while safeguarding a specific image of their business. We can understand parents seeking to protect their children from this by any means necessary.

But the viciousness of the world is the viciousness of people. We dodge our complicity in it when we leave parents believing their only option is to change bodies and not minds. Should our society ever fully live up to its stated commitment to disability rights, parents of dwarf children will worry about their chances of success and acceptance no more than the parents of left-handed children do today. Only then will they be able to opt for or against major surgeries like limb-lengthening free from social pressure.

This requires everyone – those of us with and without children – to ask ourselves tough questions. Questions like, would my best friend laugh at dwarf-tossing? Would the guys I hang out with shout at a dwarf in the street? Would I be brave enough to call them out on it? Have I ever accused someone of having a Napoleon complex? Is my daughter the type to trash other girls' bodies? Does she look up to those who do? When was the last time I criticised someone's physique? What do I think of when I think of a 'freak'? And in the nature versus nurture debate, we must stop saying 'nurture' and start saying 'culture' because it takes more than one set of parents to change the world.

This is why I run diversity workshops for teachers and parents of preschoolers. In preschool, we can take advantage of children's innocence of social markers. They are the most likely to accept the explanation the doctor gave my parents shortly after my birth: 'We're all different, Emily's difference is just more noticeable'. This is an opportunity for promoting revolutionary thinking. Differences can indeed be explained in the same matter-of-fact way we explain left-handedness. This calls for including minority conditions in every anatomy lesson. Instead of teaching bodies that fall within the norm as the rule and those that fall outside as rule-breakers, it's far more accurate to speak of any bodily variations as we do variations in hair colour, e.g.: 'Most people in the world have black hair, but many don't'. 'Most men are taller than women, but many aren't'. 'Most women have breasts, but many don't'. 'Most people walk to get around, but many don't'. Describing never-before-seen bodies and body parts as 'different' or even 'extraordinary' and never 'funny-looking' or 'ugly' can help shed light on the fact – still widely considered a radical notion – that a healthy body does not have to look 'normal'.

For every fairy tale or freak show representation of dwarfism kids will encounter – and they undoubtedly will – they need to see realistic portrayals of disabilities that offer up facts and information as early as possible. Unfortunately, the best, most comprehensive picture book on achondroplasia that accompanied me from kindergarten through primary school, *Thinking Big* by photojournalist Susan Kuklin, has been out of print for decades. I cling to my two tattered copies like precious artefacts. Recent picture books on dwarfism are well-intentioned but fall short of being informative, lacking in facts about everyday life with dwarfism and too often featuring cartoon illustrations that offer children no true markers of any diagnosis they are likely to see in real life. Their slapdash quality reflects the meagre funding such publications tend to receive. There are currently far better picture books and resources on other disabilities, which I embrace, since intersectional teaching is key to fostering empathy. After reading *Zoom!* by Robert Munsch and *Not So Different* by Shane Burcaw, the little ones in my life genuinely envy that I got to use a wheelchair for 2 years and dream of one day owning an electric one.

Indeed, alongside their thirst for information, children are keen to celebrate disabled culture when the adults around them are serious about it. Learning to finger spell in their local sign language boosts children's learning of the spoken and written alphabet while opening a window into the world's many Deaf cultures. As disability activist Jessica Kellgren-Fozard advises, such knowledge is enlightenment, and it lowers the chance she'll be approached by a child who asks, 'Why do you flap your hands around?' (Kellgren-Fozard, 2023).

I encourage parents who turn on the TV or buy tickets to non-disabled sporting events to pursue disabled events with the same frequency. The United States has long done a paltry job of promoting such events in contrast to Canada, Australia and the United Kingdom, where hours of television coverage of the Paralympics of 2012 was 100 times that of the United States Things improved at the next Paralympic Games, but in the age of YouTube, no one has any more excuses. Videos of the World Dwarf Games are just as easy to find as video tutorials on constructing Edwardian corsets and clips of a teenage Jodie Foster singing in French. Unfortunately, the YouTube algorithm too often recommends 'midgets chasing camels' and other degrading media, but this problem plagued broadcast television long before the internet got going.

As they grow and start to first observe, experience or tend towards bullying, we must teach kids about the human rights abuses of the past and present. And we must teach them it doesn't have to be this way. After all, left-handed people were – and, in some countries today, still are – forced to use their right. During the seminars I taught about dwarfism and limb-lengthening to pupils ages 13–18, I would write the following quotation on the chalkboard, paraphrased from a French magazine article in which I was featured as a child:

> Society does not accept physical differences easily. Without a doubt, that is society's fault. But who should change? Society or the dwarf? For the dwarf to change, she must undergo years of painful surgeries and intensive physical therapy, risking many complications. For society to change, it must alter its way of thinking. Who suffers more in the change? Which change is harder to achieve?

Every single one of the classes I taught gave the same answer. To the first question: The dwarf suffers more. To the second question: Society is harder to change. I told them that I want to change both.

Anyone who has had limb-lengthening faces the temptation to embrace the privileges their altered body is afforded and ditch their dwarf identity altogether. After all, it can be draining. A friend of mine was recently commiserating with me over the emotional toll of thinking about your identity in terms of polarising political debates. 'Sometimes you just don't want to dig into issues that affect you personally', she said.

'Yep', I agreed. 'Like wondering if and how many of my friends would still be friends with me if I hadn't had limb-lengthening'.

My friend paused in shock and then asked, 'Do you *have to* wonder about that? I mean, you can't change the past, so why bother yourself with that question at all?'

'You're right, I don't have to. It's a hard thing to think about. But society should, right? If anything is going to change?'

'Oh, yes. That's true. Society has to. Definitely'.

'But who's going to ask that question if I don't?'

This is why I lead discussions in classrooms and online, confronting all hierarchies based on our delusions of normalcy. Dwarf activists who can and do opt for limb-lengthening – whether in the form of surgery or that newfangled drug vosoritide – must continue to advocate for better accessibility on behalf of all dwarfs, including those whose bodies are not conducive to such treatments. Dwarf advocacy organisations in many countries have made great strides in increasing opportunities for living independently, but we cannot forget people with disabilities living in institutions where dwarfs were once regularly abandoned shortly after birth. German disability rights activist Raúl Krauthausen, who has osteogenesis imperfecta and lives independently, has reported on and even gone undercover in such institutions to reveal a disturbing lack of respect for boundaries and self-determination (Aguayo-Krauthausen, 2016).

We would be lying if any of us claimed that having a certain disability rid us of the impulse to notice other body types we rarely see. Having endured drunken men eyeballing my scars in a subway station didn't stop me from registering the bright crimson mark on the cheek of a woman standing next to me in another subway station the next day. But I kept my scars because I am proud of them and because I wanted to remember my commitment to changing my body and our culture, as well as the biases our culture has ingrained in me. It must accept me – scars and all – along with everyone else whose difference is harmless to everyone but feared by so many.

Just as body positive movements should never stall at helping only non-disabled women and girls, our call for broadening beauty standards and romantic ideals must join activism on behalf of all bodies that have been ridiculed or sidelined: from disabled, transgender, non-binary and intersex bodies to those denigrated by racism, colourism and ageism. We must speak out against dwarf-tossing in North America and against the persecution of people with albinism in Tanzania. We must link the lookism that laughs at, pities, harasses and fetishises dwarf bodies to all forms of lookism that create hierarchies of human biology. A 2014 study of popular online dating sites in Boston, New York, Chicago and Seattle that found white people, Black men, Asian women, educated men and very young women are considered far more conventionally attractive by site users than Black women, Asian men, women with higher education and women over 18 (Robinson, 2018). Many of us with dwarfism belong to many of these groups. Any one of us can attest that our mainstream beauty standards hurt more people than they help.

Whenever a member of a minority declares, 'I want to see people on TV who look like me', we must remind the media that everyone deserves to see and benefits from seeing every kind of body there is. If we must have people with dwarfism on reality TV and in fantasy films, then we must also see dwarfs as newsreaders and game show hosts, in sitcoms and dramas, in romcoms and thrillers, playing the leads and the heartthrobs and kick-ass heroes and the bella donnas. More than once. And when we succeed, we must keep the questions going: What about leads with muscle spasticity? What about Down syndrome? What about scars, burns and vitiligo? What about women with facial hair? What about every physical marker of every ethnic group deemed inferior anywhere on the planet today? We deserve to see beauty ideals that include the full variety of human bodies with such regularity that we can come to expect nothing less.

Liberating our standards of beauty must go hand in hand with liberating our measures of success. Sharing my story has attuned to me to how limb-lengthening often ends up in the news stories that contribute to the ableist trend of paying attention to disabled people only in instances of exceptional achievement. Human interest sections regularly feature pieces about someone with a disability who defied expectations and participated in the non-disabled Olympics or hiked all the national parks. At the personal level, these stories can be profoundly meaningful to the individuals at the heart of them. But the public has used them for far too long as nothing more than inspiration porn: inspiring non-disabled people to count their blessings and make changes in their own personal lives to face more challenges, never inspiring them to work to change the wider world to include disabled people as anything more than limiting stereotypes. You can tell it's inspiration porn when no one is listening to what the disability rights movement has to say.

Every sort of disabled body can and should revolutionise how we define success. 'Bad-ass strength' and 'hardcore endurance' should describe skills for not just marathon-running and rock-climbing but physical therapy and pain management. In the upper and middle classes, 'being busy' is considered a status symbol, evoking jet-setting and managing a hefty schedule of long work hours, childcare, exercise and self-improvement like cooking classes and kickboxing. This image of success needs to broaden to include the boss skills needed for managing any of the above alongside multiple therapies, medical check-ups, the accompanying paperwork and time spent lying down flat to give your back and joints much-needed rest.

Such widening of perspective will only help our calls for rest, support and accessibility in the form of expanded sick days, social benefits, healthcare and counselling centres, all of which are necessary if we are to achieve equal opportunities for those with every sort of disability of all socio-economic realities. We must simultaneously call for media portrayals and cultural values to deconstruct the shame attached to social support that too often scares those in need of it from requesting it. When 6-year-old Jennifer Keelan-Chaffins joined the 1990 protest for the Americans with Disabilities Act and hauled her disabled body up 83 stone steps to the entrance of the US Capitol, she did it to prove the necessity of installing elevators. Not to prove that any wheelchair user could crawl to the top if they were just tough enough to try and train for it. Heroes, after all, are those who fight for justice, not personal glory.

Equal opportunities for everyone are a lot to aspire to. It was unthinkable for most of human history. But then again, laminectomies and limb-lengthening were unthinkable for most of human history. Surely social progress is as attainable as technological progress. Only in a society free of bigotry against any body types will anyone be able to make decisions about body-altering procedures freely.

At this time, writing in 2024, minority rights movements are receiving more attention across the globe than ever before. Passionate discussions of underrepresentation have broken out of the margins and into the mainstream discourse, alongside comprehensive studies of crimes committed by powerful institutions: from the royal houses of Europe and other beneficiaries of colonialism to the media to the churches to the universities to the medical establishment. It's not entirely new. Today's activists stand on the shoulders of the civil rights, women's rights, gay rights, disability rights and anti-colonial activists, who in turn stood on the shoulders of countless protestors and thinkers. But today's activists are more aware of intersectional discrimination than any of our predecessors. Never before have so many governments had so many anti-discrimination laws protecting so many different minorities simultaneously. Never before have we had so many opportunities to utilise someone's understanding of one injustice to enlighten them to others.

However, there has also been horrifying backlash to all of this. Outright hate and death threats for any minority are but a Google search away. Populist politicians have won elections in the world's largest democracies by convincing voters that the biggest problems today are the whiny minorities, predatory freaks and the woke mobs. The sheer volume of the vitriol, let alone the violence, makes it easy to collapse into despair about humanity.

But to give up hope or to downplay the dream of true equality as naive is to insult the memory of everyone who made the wonderful life I have possible. I've grown up in one of the safest times in human history to be a person living with dwarfism. We did not get to this point by merely evolving like some flower of progress that was planted and set to blossom in the 21st century after millennia of infanticide and abuse. I live in Berlin, a city that in my own relatives' lifetime passed ordinances to have people like me murdered in an attempt to wipe us out forever. The city is proof of humanity's capacity to change for better and for worse. My very existence here and the opportunities I have had are the result of dauntingly hard work done by those who did not give in to cynicism. I owe it to them – to every family member, teacher, doctor, activist and to every dwarf victim of the Nazis, to every dwarf baby abandoned in an institution or circus, to every dwarf adult traded among the Early Modern aristocracy as a pet, to every dwarf child thrown off a cliff in Ancient Sparta – to enjoy the freedom, safety and love I have and to use it to work for a fairer world.

References

Abramovitch, S. (2016, August 25). Little people, big woes in Hollywood: Low pay, degrading jobs and a tragic death. *The Hollywood Reporter* [online]. https://www.hollywoodreporter.com/movies/movie-features/little-people-actors-actresses-low-pay-degrading-jobs-tragedy-922261/. Accessed on May 27, 2023.

Adelson, B. M. (2005). *Dwarfism: Medical and psychosocial aspects of profound short stature.* The Johns Hopkins University Press.

Aguayo-Krauthausen, R. (2016, September 22). Raúl Krauthausen lebt für fünf Tagen undercover in Pflegeheim. *JETZT* [online]. https://www.jetzt.de/teilhabegesetz/raul-krauthausen-lebt-fuer-fuenf-tage-undercover-im-pflegeheim. Accessed on June 03, 2023.

Allanson, J. E., & Hall, J. G. (1986, January). Obstetric and gynecologic problems in women with chondrodystrophies. *Obstetrics & Gynecology, 67*(1), 74–78.

Arnold, J., & Klein, B. (2015). *Life is short (no pun intended): Love, laughter and learning to enjoy every moment.* Howard Books.

Chester, N. (2015, March 30). Life can be tough for LGBT little people: An interview with a gay dwarf. *Vice* [online]. https://www.vice.com/en/article/7bdp3z/lgbt-little-people-729. Accessed on May 02, 2023.

Cokely, R. (2017, September 23). Little people, big depression. *Medium* [online]. https://rebecca-cokley.medium.com/little-people-big-depression-2ba274fbff68. Accessed on June 23, 2023.

Coontz, S. (2000). *The way we never were: American families and the nostalgia trap.* Basic Books.

Davies, J. H., Child, J., Freer, J., & Storr, H. L. (2023). Inequalities in the assessment of childhood short stature. *British Journal of General Practice, 73*(729), 150–151.

Gerson, M. N. (2014, 29 July). The challenges of having sex as a little person. *The Atlantic* [online]. https://www.theatlantic.com/health/archive/2014/07/the-challenges-of-having-sex-as-a-little-person/374647/. Accessed on June 09, 2023.

Harrell, E. (2021). *Crime against persons with disabilities, 2009–2019 – Statistical table.* Bureau of Justice Statistics, U.S. Department of Justice [online]. https://bjs.ojp.gov/library/publications/crime-against-persons-disabilities-2009-2019-statistical-tables. Accessed on June 15, 2023.

Kellgren-Fozard, J. (2023, April 3). Why are you flapping your hands around? Jessica Kellgren-Fozard [online video]. https://www.youtube.com/watch?v=KZFh69uME7M. Accessed on June 29, 2023.

Robinson, M. (2018, April 10). Dude, she's (exactly 25 percent) out of your league. *The Atlantic* [online]. https://www.theatlantic.com/science/archive/2018/08/online-dating-out-of-your-league/567083/. Accessed on June 12, 2023.

Epilogue

Erin Pritchard (Senior Lecturer in Disability Studies)
Liverpool Hope University, UK

How It Started

From sculpture to podcasts, this book demonstrates the various ways advocates raise awareness about dwarfism. Adelson (2005a) points out that general society, including the disability community, is not fully aware of the push people with dwarfism are trying to make to challenge and change cultural representations of the condition. The initial aim of the book was to respond to the scarce literature on dwarfism in disability arts. As numerous authors have pointed out, dwarfism is a disability, and thus disability arts need to reflect on how it can be inclusive for people with dwarfism. Amanda Cachia eloquently demonstrates that disability arts can be empowering. Both Cachia and Robson show how it can serve as a platform to showcase our spatial experiences. However, as Tamm Reynolds shows, people with dwarfism can feel out of place within this sector of the industry. For example, Reynold's chapter demonstrates how the Shaw Trust deems Warwick Davis to be an influential disabled person, but within the dwarfism community, not everyone would agree. Furthermore, Steph Robson also shows that other disabled people can undermine the aim of raising awareness about dwarfism. Thus, there appears to be a hierarchy of impairments, and as a result, the book was expanded to go beyond the subject. As Robson pointed out, it allows people with dwarfism to engage in the arts on their own terms.

Dwarf Pride

Numerous chapters show how representations of dwarfism continue to be shaped by average-sized people. Creating our own representation of dwarfism is an empowering process and a step towards fostering dwarf pride. Part of dwarf pride is about challenging stereotypes to provide a more realistic representation that can elevate the social standing of people with dwarfism. We need to create our own identity, a true to life identity that we can be proud of. This pride needs to shun pity and instead celebrate our achievements that are not *in spite* of our dwarfism but instead are *despite* the ableist structures and attitudes that we experience daily. In turn, this will provide a better social standing for people with dwarfism.

The contributors to the book should be admired for their work. Nic Noviki demonstrates an immense pride in being a little person, which he refers to as 'dwarf pride'. Exploring why difference is good and should be celebrated challenges height altering treatments, which Emily Sullivan-Sanford and Alice Lambert both explore but with differing opinions. Lambert uses performance art to challenge height altering treatments, while Sullivan-Sanford is frank about not regretting her choice to undergo leg-lengthening, but instead uses it as a basis to question society's acceptance of dwarfism. While Sullivan-Sanford chose to undergo limb-lengthening treatment, and we should recognise a person's free will to do so, we must look at how dwarf pride is undermined in a world that reveres tallness. As all chapters have shown, there is a lot of dwarf pride being shared in various ways. However, this pride which challenges dominant representations and ideas about dwarfism must be given more attention.

Working in the Entertainment Industry

The experiences of those working in the entertainment industry provide a nuanced account of who is responsible for perpetuating the metanarrative of dwarfism. In the entertainment industry, these include writers and producers, who have been in control of how people with dwarfism are represented on screen and stage. However, as this book shows, there are numerous people with dwarfism, who are utilising an array of ways to challenge dominant ideas of dwarfism. Both Reynolds and Lambert challenge representations of dwarfism in the pantomime. This is important to highlight because in the United Kingdom, it is often assumed that people with dwarfism rely on the pantomime as a form of employment (Grant, 2017; Pritchard, 2023).

It is not easy to say no to a role when people with dwarfism already face employment discrimination in other occupations. As Sam Drummond shows, he experienced numerous incidents of employment discrimination due to his dwarfism yet never restored to midget entertainment. Furthermore, Lambert makes it clear that even if she was struggling financially, she would still not resort to midget entertainment. Thus, society must not assume that midget entertainment is some sort of security net for people with dwarfism. Furthermore, while all of the contributors have an impressive educational background, as Woodburn and Lambert demonstrate, numerous medical procedures impacted their educational opportunities.

Declining a role in a film or television show can have huge consequences, both financially and for the actor's career. Declining a role in a film or television show does not automatically mean that the actor will be out of work, but it is a risky decision. Actors with dwarfism deserve the same opportunities as any other actor, but that does not mean that midget entertinment 'is a job for them'. Actors in this book have worked hard to get where they are today. Those who are declining roles demonstrate how unacceptable numerous people with dwarfism find particular representations of the condition. Many of them have gone through college to learn performance techniques, instead of thinking that somehow their dwarfism gives them the right and an easy root into the industry. Furthermore, as

Lambert points out, many midget entertainers lack an educational background in drama and instead rely solely on using their dwarfism to fulfil roles. Thus, while we should also be advocating for increased educational opportunities that provide people with dwarfism the tools needed for the industry, we also need to recognise that it still does not mean that they will be successful.

Creating Our Own Representations

While actors with dwarfism are making great strides in changing how dwarfism is depicted on screen and stage, others are creating change in other ways. Drummond demonstrates how working in radio and later writing his memories helps to challenge misconceptions about dwarfism. Furthermore, media creators, such as Kara B Ayers, Steph Robson and Jillian Ilana, are raising awareness that writers and producers should also be taking notice of. While Ayers rightly points out that social media platforms are rife with material that mocks people with dwarfism, we need to be using these platforms to raise awareness. Thus, the message entwined within all of these chapters is that people with dwarfism need to be actively making their own space within all spaces that tell us that we do not belong. As Robson notes, we need to 'take space' to show our lived experiences. This is not an easy task, given that our daily experiences are mired by unwanted attention that signifies that we do not belong.

Contributors have shown the importance of actively creating their own representations as opposed to abiding by preconceived ableist ideas of dwarfism. Robson strengthened this call by arguing for people with dwarfism to be offered more opportunities in disability arts. Noviki is answering this call by providing people with a great opportunity for more people with dwarfism to be challenged in creating their own representations. Furthermore, Simon Minty demonstrates how comedy does not have to be off limits to be people with dwarfism. Creating our own representations challenges the belief that we have to abide by problematic stereotypes and representations to be employed. However, this requires those who work in the entertainment industry to have the right tools, including a good educational background. Many of the contributors in this book show that they have a good educational background, that they have the ability, the talent, the imagination to create more positive representations and the confidence to challenge producers and writers.

On Editing

Editing chapters and interviewing contributors has been a cathartic process. As a person with dwarfism who is often exposed to numerous derogatory representations of the condition, I have found it wonderful to engage with so many people with dwarfism who are pushing for a more positive representation of our condition. I hope that others reading this book have come away with the same feeling. I also hope that those who may have never questioned stereotypical representations of people with dwarfism now realise that these are not universally accepted within the dwarfism community.

The decision to encourage advocates to write their own chapter provided them with the ability to share their views and experiences, with little input from me as the editor. As Drummond eloquently explains that even with the best intentions, average-sized writers can misinterpret our voices. While I have dwarfism, I still felt that the decision gave them more of a voice. This has allowed them to share what they have deemed important and the achievements they are proud of. It also means that terminology may sometimes differ, but this reflects their sociocultural background and beliefs. Where this has not been possible, I have tried to limit my input and used prompts to engage with their work and highlight their achievements. As a result, in some cases, I have had to reflect on my own beliefs and ensure that these do not interfere with any of the chapters.

One belief I have always held is that people who partake in midget entertainment are largely responsible for how dwarfism is represented and subsequently perceived. This was an opinion also evident in Drummond, Lambert and Minty's chapters. Drummond clearly shows how he is treated in society is reflective of how dwarfism is depicted in the media. Furthermore, as Minty pointed out, those who hire themselves out have a choice. It is interesting to note, however, that not all authors agreed with this notion. For example, both Danny Woodburn and Nic Noviki blame writers and producers. Working in the industry, they were able to demonstrate some of the difficulties people with dwarfism experience. While Woodburn and Noviki attest that the blame lies with writers and producers, we should also consider why they continue to perpetuate the metanarrative of dwarfism. Yet, as Lambert and Minty's chapters show, those who agree to derogatory roles aid in encouraging average-sized creators to push the metanarrative of dwarfism. The more people who say no to roles that dehumanise and mock our condition, the more chance we have of changing how we are represented. We need to send a collective message to writers and producers that particular representations of dwarfism should be assigned to the history books. However, we do not fully understand the circumstances of these entertainers. As Woodburn explains, entertainment is a hard industry to make it in and to remain financially stable; many actors rely on second jobs, which people with dwarfism cannot always fulfil. Thus, while we need to push for more positive representations of dwarfism, we also need to advocate for better education and employment opportunities.

Where to Go From Here

Minty, Noviki and Robson are providing the tools and support for others to challenge the metanarrative of dwarfism. Yet, there are still people with dwarfism choosing to engage in derogatory roles, which impacts the social standing of all people with dwarfism. It is important to point out that while people with dwarfism do experience employment discrimination, these roles are still a choice. However, it is a choice that is being offered by average-sized creators. While all of these chapters show that there is progress being made about equality for people with dwarfism, as Angela van Etten rightly points out, there is still a long way to go. Producers, writers and creators need to engage with people with dwarfism to understand why it is important to create more authentic representations of dwarfism. As with other minority groups, media services need to reflect on historical representations of dwarfism and how they contribute to our unequal social standing.

While some of the contributors are part of associations for people with dwarfism, and in the case of van Etten have acted as president of the world's largest association for people with dwarfism, it is interesting to note how the majority are pushing for equality without support from associations. Associations for people with dwarfism often claim that they push for equality, yet this is not always evident. In the case of Lambert, the association she was part of was not very proactive in pushing against derogatory roles. Thus, what are associations doing or what can they do to push for dwarf pride? Associations for people with dwarfism could benefit from engaging with the various artists and media creators within this book. Associations need to be open about collaboration and be willing to learn from individuals with dwarfism.

This book is made up of contributors both men and women, which challenges the stereotypical representation of male races of dwarfs. Reynolds's chapter also provides an intersectional representation of dwarfism. Reynold's engagement with drag performances aids in demonstrating nuanced ways of challenging the metanarrative of dwarfism. Furthermore, through the use of memoir, Drummond provides an insight into the life of a person with dwarfism from a single-parent family. However, a limitation of this book is the diverse racial experiences of dwarfism. The intention was to include a diverse range of voices. Adverts calling for authors were placed on various social media pages for people with dwarfism, including the *LPA Dwarf Artist Coalition*. I, as the editor, also contacted various people with dwarfism working in the arts and beyond. Many of the contributors were part of associations for people with dwarfism, which are predominantly made up of white, middle-class people with dwarfism (Adelson, 2005b). Furthermore, when researching artists with dwarfism, most that I came across identified as white. However, there are people with dwarfism from different racial backgrounds who should be noted for their contributions, for example, Aubrey Smalls, an actor and film-maker with dwarfism, whose work highlights his experiences as a person with dwarfism. Thus, there needs to be further consideration of the intersecting identities of people with dwarfism and the importance of raising awareness and fostering dwarf pride. As Steph Robson rightly points out, we need to ensure that all sections of the dwarfism community are included.

References

Adelson, B. (2005a). The changing lives of archetypal 'curiosities' – And echoes of the past. *Disability Studies Quarterly, 25*(3), 1–13.

Adelson, B. (2005b). *Dwarfism: Medical and psychosocial aspects of profound short stature.* The John Hopkins University Press.

Grant, E. (2017). I have dwarfism, and no I don't 'do panto' – Casting people like me in stereotypical roles is damaging and insulting. *The Independent* [online]. https://www.independent.co.uk/voices/Pantomime-roles-dwarfism-acting-theatre-dwarf-people-stereotypes-casting-do-panto-damaging-insulting-a8107221.html. Accessed on February 27, 2024.

Pritchard, E. (2023). *Midgetism: The exploitation and discrimination of people with dwarfism.* Routledge.

Index

Ableism, 151
Ableist curator, 12–15
Ableist portrayals reduction without censorship, 128
Abnormally Funny People, 90, 92, 95
Achondroplasia, 79, 149–150
Act of judging, 28–29
Advertising dwarfs, 56–57
Advocacy, 2–3
   specialist, 107
Aesthetic encounters, 30–31
Ain, Michael, 79, 150
Aladdin in Dorset, 55–56
Always Looking Up, 132–134
Ambulatory automatism, 21–22
American Association of People With Disabilities (AAPD), 136
Americans with Disabilities Act (1990), 22, 132, 158–159
Americans with Disabilities Act Accessibility Guidelines (ADAAG), 117
Angela Muir Van Etten blog: A voice for people with dwarfism & disability, 112–113
Annenberg Inclusion Initiative, 101
ANSI Committee, 116–117
Anti-ableism, 121–122
Architectural barriers, 115
Are You Afraid of the Dark? (1990–1996), 84
Artistic work, 23
Artworks, 25–26
Associations, 165
Automatisme Ambulatoire: Hysteria, Imitation, Performance, 21–22

Average-height (AH) people, 121–123
Awareness-raising, 38–41

Bad-ass strength, 158
Bardot, Midgitte, 63
   adoption of queer spaces, 66–67
   using drag to challenge midgetism, 67–73
   performances, 64–66
Barrister, 107
Black Lives Matter movement, 55–56
Brachyolmia, 11
British Vogue, 132–133
Broke, 140–144
Building coalitions, 117–118

Center for Independent Living (CIL), 110
Cheyenne, Sofiya, 105
Christian Law Association (CLA), 110
Civil rights, 116
Classical impairments, 95
Collective voice, 4
Comedy, 95–97
Competence, 117
Computer-generated imagery (CGI), 78
Confrontational inertness, 31
Conspiratorial power, 30
Contemporary exhibitions, 19
Corban rule, 15–16
Cornflakes, 77–78
Cranston, Bryan, 85–86
Creative activist, 42–43
Creative Development Fellowship, 43
Crenna, Richard, 77–78
Crip Camp, 133
Cripping up, 85
Crocodile Dundee, 142

Cultural sensitivities, 55–56
Cyrano, 92

Danish Dwarf Association, The, 4
Dave the Dwarf personality, 116
Davis, Warwick, 39–40, 70, 72
Developmental years, 108–109
Disability, 63, 90
  aesthetics, 22, 27–28
  community, 161
  social-relational framework of, 26–29
Disability advocacy on social media, 126–128
  leveraging audience for disability advocacy, 126–127
  prioritising quality over quantity in media representation, 128
  unpacking inspiration porn, 127
Disability arts, 3–4, 161
  and advocacy, 2–3
Disability equality
  avoiding stereotypes, 78–82
  getting roles, 77–78
  Paying the Price, 83–85
  Seinfeld, 82–83
  Songs to Grow On, 76
  Woodburn Ratio, 85–87
Disability Rights Education and Defense Fund (DREDF), 117–118
Disability Rights Movement, 135
Disabled movement, 22
Disabled Parenting Project, The, 125
Disabled people, 101
Disaboom, 123–124
Discrimination and acceptance from within dwarfism community, 44–45
Disney+, 55–56
Dobbs v. Jackson Women's Health Organization, 135
Doctors (2023), 40
Down Syndrome, 149
Drag performances, 69
Dwarf, 5

Dwarf culture, 37, 46
  making case for, 46–48
Dwarf entertainer, 56–57
Dwarf people, 37–38
Dwarf pride, 161–162
Dwarf tossing, 115
Dwarfism, 1, 11, 26, 51, 65, 67, 81, 89, 121–122, 131, 139, 145, 161, 164
  in 3D, 29–30
  Ableist curator, 12–15
  Abnormally Funny People, 92–95
  advocacy, 107
  awareness-raising, 38–41
  background as content creator with, 122–124
  combating negative encounters, 111–115
  and comedy, 95–97
  curating and disrupting movement, 17–22
  developmental years, 108–109
  discrimination and acceptance from within dwarfism community, 44–45
  disrupting mobility and vision, 15–17
  dwarf culture, 46
  effective advocacy principles, 115–118
  identifying identity gap between educating and objectification, 38
  intentionality behind sharing personal experiences, 125–126
  legal training and career, 109–111
  life lesson, 98–100
  lived experience, 37
  navigating local and national communities, politics and gatekeepers in arts in United Kingdom, 45
  new views, 22–23
  participatory artist and creative activist, 42–43

participatory engagement, 43–44
practising as practitioner, 45–46
sharing glimpses into life as mother with, 125–126
struggle to articulate and accept identity and agency, 41–42
Dwarfs Sports Association UK (DSAUK), 4
Dwarfs: Not A Fairy Tale, 150

Easterseals Disability Film Challenge, 102–103
  goal, 104–105
  little people and comedy, 103–104
Editing, 163–164
Editor, 107
Effective advocacy principles, 115–118
Elite actors, 76
Elmer the Patchwork Elephant, 139
Entertain-Ment, 56–57
Entertainment industry, 162–163
Epilepsy, 21–22
Equity, 58
Ethics of Dwarfism and Humour, 40
Europe, 105
Experiencing bullying, 52

Family Guy, 95
Farley Brothers, 101
Figurative sculpture, 31
Films, 75
Fire Island, 151
504 Sit-ins of 1977, 133
Flesh of the World, The, 20
Forces for Change, 132–133
Freak show, 54
French film comedy, 21–22

Game of Thrones series, 90–92
Girl power voices, 151
'Girl Talk', 134
Gogglebox, 90, 99
Great Comic Relief Bake Off, The (2013), 40
Great Curiosities, 111

Green M&M's scenario, 87
Gunslinger robot, 78

Half Monty, The, 98
Hardcore endurance, 158
HelloLittleLady.com, 37, 42
Historical treatments for dwarfism, 60
Hollyoaks (2023), 40
Hollywood Reporter, The, 149–150
Honey, I've Joined the Big Top, 80
Honey. I Shrunk the Kids (Television series), 80
Hope and Faith, 81
Hysteria, 21–22

Identity gap between educating and objectification, 38
Industrial materials, 15
Inspiration porn, 127
Intersectionality, 149–150
Intersubjectivity, 29

Jerk (2019-present), 94–95
Jingle All the Way (1996), 81
Jones, James Earl, 77–78

Lansbury, Angela, 78
Larsen's syndrome, 107
Last Leg, The (2012-present), 94–95
Legal training and career, 109–111
Legal writer, 107
LGBTQIA+, 64
Life's Too Short (Davis), 39, 70
Limb-lengthening, 145–146, 148–149, 153
  characterising, 147
  social benefits, 146
'Little Big Woman: Condescension', 25–26
  dwarfism in 3D, 29–30
  oppositional gaze, 30–33
  social-relational framework of disability, 26–29

Little people and comedy, 103–104
Little People of America (LPA), 4, 8, 115, 117, 131–132
Little People of America convention, 14–15, 152–153
Little People of Canada, 4
Little People of Ireland, 4
Little People of New Zealand, 4
Little People UK (LPUK), 4
Little People's Research Fund, 149
Living in Oblivion, 90–91
Lost Voice Guy, 94–95
Loudermilk (2018–2020), 105
LPA Dwarf Artist Coalition, 165

Mary Poppins Returns, 52
Media, 2, 8, 55
Medical model, 26
Metanarrative of disability, 2
Metanarrative of dwarfism, 2
Midget, 127
Midget entertainers, 2
Midget entertainment, 1, 68–69, 164
Midget tossing, 2, 4
Midgetism, 67–73
Mobility
 disrupting, 15–17
 limitations, 95
Murder, She Wrote, 78

Netflix, 55–56
Networked individualism, 123
No Limits, 141
Non-disabled creators, 126
'Normal' up and down movement, 16
Normalising procedures, 60
Notice of Proposed Rulemaking (NPRM), 117

Object–subject positioning, 31
Online dwarfism communities, 126–127

Oppositional gaze, 30–33
Oppression Olympics, 151
Osteogenesis Imperfecta (OI), 122
Outsider perspectives, 23
Outstanding Alumni Achievement Award, 75
Overcoming disability, 126

Pantomime, 53–54
Participatory artist, 42–43
Participatory arts, 37
Participatory engagement, 43–44
Participatory movement, 20–21
Passions (1999–2007), 84
'Pathologised' body, 21–22
People with dwarfism, 1, 47, 56, 80, 165
Perfect show broadcast, 94–95
Performance art, 60
Personal evolution as content creator and researcher, 122–125
 background as content creator with dwarfism, 122–124
 impact on dispelling stereotypes and fostering understanding, 126
 journey as researcher studying disability portrayals in media, 124–125
Picket Fences (1992–1996), 80–81
Planes, Trains & Automobiles (1987), 102
Podcasts, 131
 advocating through, 134–136
 In the Beginning–In the Search for Equality, 132–134
Political freak, 63–64, 72
Presley's movement, 22
Project Runway, 132–133
Pros and Cons (1991–1992), 77–78
Pseudoachondroplasia, 139
Psycho-emotional disablism, 63, 69

Index

Queer spaces, adoption of, 66–67

Radio City Rockettes, 84–85
Ramp Up, 141
Realpolitik of disability, 25–26, 29
Relational disability aesthetics, 25–27, 29
Representations, 163
Restricted Growth Association (RGA), 4
Roe v. Wade and *Planned Parenthood v. Casey*, 135
'Roll You Home' blog, 124
Russell Silver Syndrome, 41

Screen Actors Guild (SAG), 75
Section 504 of the Rehabilitation Act (1973), 132
Seinfeld, 82–83
Self-advocacy, 107
Self-awareness, 122
Self-reflexivity, 122
Sensory loss, 95
Sexuality, 63, 81
Shaw Trust, 72
Short Statured People of Australia (SSPA), 4
Short Statured Scotland (SSS), 4
Silk Stalkings: Passion and the Palm Beach Detectives, 79
Sky Television, 92
Small Teen, Bigger World (2011), 41–42
Snow White and the Seven Dwarfs, 54–56
Social media, 59–60, 121
    disability advocacy on social media, 126–128
    intersection of personal experiences and academic pursuits, 125
    personal evolution as content creator and researcher, 122–125
    reduction of ableist portrayals without censorship, 128
    sharing glimpses into life as mother with dwarfism, 125–126
Social-relational framework of disability, 26–29
    relational disability aesthetics, 27–29
Soda Jerk, 77
Solicitor, 107
Something has to be done about this!, 115
Songs to Grow On, 76
Spatial experiences of dwarfism, 12
Spectatorship, 21–22
Spider-Man: Across the Spider-Verse (2023), 101
Spondyloepiphyseal Dysplasia Congenita (SEDc), 84
Stanchions (tool), 16–17
Star Wars, 89–90
Stir Crazy (1980), 102
Strictly Come Dancing contestant, 40
Subjectivity, 29
Suit fillers, 53, 61

Taking Space, 47
Television shows, 75
Tin Drum and *Even Dwarfs Started Off Small, The*, 151
Total Recall (1990), 81
Trading Places (1983), 102

Ultra-marginalisation, 153
Unconscious imitation, 21–22
UNION Arts, 43–44
United Kingdom, navigating local and national communities, politics and gatekeepers in arts in, 45
United Parcel Service (UPS), 84
Untitled Seatbelt series, 19–20

Venus de Milo (Greek sculpture), 27–28
Viciousness of people, 155
Viet Rock, 77
Viewer's gaze, 30

Index

Vision, disrupting, 15–17
Vogue magazines, 40, 59–60
Voices for change, 3–5
Vosoritide, 59

Walking with Giants, 4
Way We Roll, The, 90

WayFinders, 44
Wheel, The, 40
'Wheeler Mom' blog, 124
Willow, 84
Wizard of Oz, The, 89–90
Woodburn ratio, 76, 85, 87